THE 7-DAY SMOOTHIE DIET

GALVANIZED Books

This book proposes a program of diet and exercise recommendations for the reader to follow. However, you should consult a qualified medical professional (and, if you are pregnant, your ob-gyn) before starting this or any other diet or fitness program. Please seek your doctor's advice before making any decisions that affect your health or extreme changes in your diet, particularly if you suffer from any medical condition or have any symptom that may require treatment. As with any diet or exercise program, if at any time you experience discomfort, stop immediately and consult your physician.

Mention of specific companies, organizations, or authorities in this book does not imply endorsement by the author or publisher, nor does mention of specific companies, organizations, or authorities imply that they endorse this book, its author, or the publisher.

Distributed by Simon & Schuster.

ISBN 978-1-940358-20-8
Ebook ISBN 978-1-940-358-21-5

Printed in the United States of America on acid-free paper.

Design by Andy Turnbull.

THE 7-DAY SMOOTHIE DIET

Lose up to a pound a day —and sip your way to a flat belly!

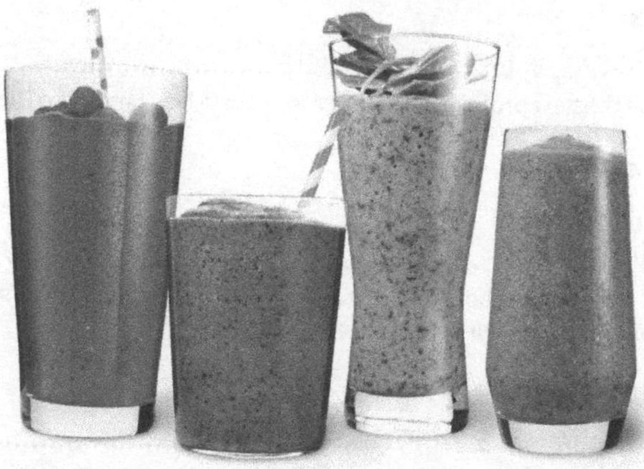

By the Editors of

Eat This, Not That!®

Contents

T0042770

THE 7-DAY SMOOTHIE DIET

INTRODUCTION

Sip into Better Health

LET ME LET YOU IN ON A LITTLE SECRET that you may find strange coming from the editor of a smoothies book:

I hate smoothies. Well, at least I did at one time.

To be honest, it's not so much the smoothie drinking I dislike as it is the smoothie cleanup: the scrubbing of the blender and wiping up of the kitchen counter afterward.

Making smoothies can leave a kitchen looking like three

preteen girls spent the afternoon engaged in that curious recent phenomenon known as "making slime." I didn't care to go through all that hassle for a liquid meal that resembled those squishy concoctions my daughter Sophia stores in every last plastic food container we own. There's not a thimbleful of white glue left in our house, but we have many, many containers of pink "unicorn slime," if you're interested.

Smoothies. What's the big deal? I prefer chewing my food to sipping it. I love to sink my teeth into a juicy steak or dive into a pizza with the works. I love the crunch of a fresh garden salad drizzled with extra virgin olive oil. Interesting flavors and textures send my taste buds dancing. You too?

Enjoying food is part of enjoying life. And who wants it liquefied? But I was missing the whole point of smoothies: A well-made smoothie is fast, filling, high nutrition in a cup. Or bowl. Drinking a smoothie can upgrade your diet and help you lose weight fast.

Hunger Busted

One day I was late for a magazine photo shoot. I had to rush out the door without breakfast. By the time I got to the studio, I was so ravenous I could have eaten, well, pink unicorn slime.

I saw one of the photo assistants chowing down on a bowl of something that looked delicious.

"What's that?" I asked.

"Smoothie bowl. Want one?"

He poured the creamy purple contents from a blender into an empty bowl and spooned banana slices, fresh blueberries, toasted coconut, chia seeds, and chopped walnuts on top. "There's granola in that box if you want it," he said.

"I'm good. This looks fantastic."

And it tasted even better. It was sweet, delicious, and thick. So thick I could stand my spoon upright in it. It felt like ... a bowl of health. And it was filling. We worked right through lunchtime and I didn't feel a hunger pang until three p.m.

That smoothie bowl, something he called the Berry Banana Walnut Bowl, was a real meal. I later learned that it also had spinach in it. Bonus! I started changing my poor opinion of smoothies.

Lately, I've been trying to eat more protein and greens and far fewer carbohydrates, especially the fast-burning, blood-sugar-boosting kind you get in cereal, bagels, pizza, spaghetti, and bread—you know, the food that's easiest to find and consume, the food that tends to be in any house where you find kids.

Protein is important for folks like me. As we age, protein becomes even more critical to support muscle growth. With each passing year in midlife, our skeletons lose muscle mass and our metabolisms slow down. If we don't keep our bodies strong with physical weight-bearing activity, if we don't eat enough protein but do continue to consume the same number of calories as we did when we were young, that lost muscle is replaced by fat. This is typically how midlife belly bulge creeps in. But even if you're naturally thin, your muscle can be replaced by fat and you become what's known as "skinny fat," which is almost as unhealthy as being "fat fat."

Whenever I feel as if I'm becoming less mindful of what I'm putting in my body, I have a system for nudging myself back on the road to healthier eating. I keep a food log for a few days. I write down everything I eat or drink in a notebook. Yeah, I know there are apps to help you do this, but the physical act of writing "6 Oreo cookies, 320 CALORIES! What were you thinkin', you dummy!" in ink is more effective for me. Been doing this for years. The notebook gives me a pretty telling picture of my regular menu. It's often the wakeup call that helps me realize that I need to stop mindlessly gobbling and start mindfully planning my meals and snacks.

My latest food diary clearly showed that I had drifted off track. I wasn't eating enough vegetables, especially leafy greens, and my diet was too rich in starchy carbs, too weak in lean proteins. What's more, I saw clearly in black and white that, for speed and convenience, most of my breakfasts were coming from a cereal box. Now, I know better. I wrote a book called *The 14-Day No Sugar Diet*. But I'm human, and humans need reminders. My food log showed that I was mixing my high-fiber muesli with Honey Bunches of Oats. Sugar city. Doesn't stick to the ribs. Actually my breakfasts made me more hungry. I found myself buying three-dollar energy bars to quell hunger pangs just before lunchtime. Hey, have you noticed how much sugar they put in most energy bars these days? It's a ton of energy.

While editing this book, I invested in a Vitamix blender and committed to drinking a breakfast smoothie every morning before work for one week, as recommended in the book's plan. It was a cool experiment with immediate benefits. For one, the smoothies replaced those sugary cereals I was eating. No, they weren't as sweet as Honey Bunches of Oats, but they were rich and filling. I wasn't hungry at 10:30

in the morning. The recipes were fun to make, and they inspired me to start concocting my own by trial and error: kale, avocado, and Cocoa Puffs? Mistake. Oats, banana, almond milk? Yum!

I started making protein shakes with chocolate-flavored pea protein powder for afternoon snacks at work at the encouragement of my colleagues, the editors at *Eat This, Not That!* and *Eatthis.com.* It's not a Yoo-hoo drink by any stretch of the imagination, but it's not half bad. You get used to the taste of plant-based protein and quickly learn how to sweeten it up a bit with frozen banana or vanilla almond milk. With a protein smoothie in my afternoon belly, I didn't need a Philly-style pretzel from Wawa or a Cliff Bar to chase the hunger away. In short order, I noticed that my pants felt looser. I had lost weight! And I found that my afternoon smoothie didn't leave me feeling sleepy.

Now I'm a convert. Smoothies make sense—for everyone. While a smoothie will never replace broiled salmon and steamed broccoli, it's certainly a fast and easy way to jam a ton of protein and vegetables into your diet and reap the nutritional bounty that you may be missing out on.

And if you want to lose pounds, drinking smoothies as meal replacements can be a convenient and delicious way to significantly reduce the consumption of processed carbohydrates and the calories that come with them, and boost sensations of satiety so you're not running to the vending machine in between meals.

Beware of Sugary Smoothies

Heads-up, folks. Not all smoothies are healthful and good for losing weight. Some pack enough sugars to rival a chocolate shake from McDonald's. And some of those sugars come from loading up the blender with lots of virtuous fruit. So be wary of what you dump into that blender. Make sure your smoothies contain protein and fiber to slow the absorption of sugars into your bloodstream, which can spike blood sugar and trigger a roller-coaster ride of carb cravings.

Concocted correctly, however, smoothies are helpful tools for cutting calories out of your daily intake. For example, smoothies made with vegetables, fruits, and fats like olive oil, dark chocolate, nuts, and seeds are an ideal delivery system for powerful antioxidants called polyphenols that have been shown to absorb fat by as much as 20 percent. Smoothies make it easy to load up on nutrients that you might not otherwise get in your diet, healthful compounds called flavonoids that fight heart disease, diabetes, and cancer; lower blood pressure; strengthen your skeleton; boost your immune system; and help you shed belly fat. Are you sure you're getting enough disease-fighting nutrients in your meals?

A friend of mine who's a real curmudgeon recently shared a quote on Facebook: "The problem with the gene pool is there's no lifeguard."

I beg to differ. You are your lifeguard—and your own best lifeguard, at that. The types (and quantities) of foods you put into your mouth directly and profoundly impact your longevity. You are what you eat, after all. And the burgeoning science of

A rich, thick smoothie for breakfast can carry you the distance to lunchtime.

epigenetics continues to demonstrate that gene expression, how genes tell cells what to do, is influenced by the lifestyle choices we make every day. Now, where do we make the greatest number of routine lifestyle choices every day? Breakfast, lunch, dinner, and snacks.

That's where smoothies can help. The more I learned about the practical health benefits of drinking nutritious smoothies, the more convinced I became that I should start incorporating them into my own diet to maintain my healthy weight and supercharge my body with immune-system-boosting nutrients I was missing. Much of that learning came from the research of the writers and editors of *Eat This, Not That!* and *Eatthis.com*, who developed this book's kick-ass seven-day program of two nutritious smoothies a day. If you believe you should be eating more vegetables and fruits or you would like to lose 10 or more pounds and feel better, I encourage you to give it a try. The plan takes only a week. (You can do anything for a week!) And I truly believe that you'll be rewarded for your efforts with a healthier, leaner body, and a more mindful approach to eating.

What Exactly is the 7-Day Smoothie Diet?

Let's begin with what the 7-Day Smoothie Diet is not: It is not a "detox" or "body cleansing" program. The idea of a detox may be trendy, but it's not based on science. Your body is a pretty miraculous machine with its own built-in detox system called the liver. Your liver does a superb job of filtering your blood and breaking down chemicals and toxins and neutralizing them. So don't be hoodwinked into

The 7-Day Smoothie

Follow these simple rules every day...

Rule 1

Drink Two Satisfying Shakes

Purpose: To quell hunger for hours without overloading you with calories and sugar. Select two smoothies from our list of recipes. The first, your breakfast smoothie, is rich in healthy fats, protein, and fiber to keep you satisfied until lunchtime. Your afternoon smoothie is lower in calories, but high in plant-based protein to knock back the craving for a late-afternoon run to the vending machine.

Rule 2

Eat Extra-Filling Food

Purpose: To fuel your body with healthy nutrition that won't leave you hungry after eating. You'll enjoy a substantial lunch and delicious full dinner using recipes from our list of selected meals to maximize nutrition and satiety.

Diet at a Glance

Rule 3

Smack Down Hunger Pangs with Cravings Crushers

Purpose: To learn techniques to gain control over emotional eating. Cravings Crushers are simple, proven tricks you can use whenever you get a hankering for a sweet or find yourself reaching for a between-meal snack just because it's there. These physical and mental distractions will help you to break the cycle of mindless eating. You'll master them in no time.

Rule 4

Get Moving!

Purpose: To rise out of a sedentary position and become active and energetic again. You don't have to join a gym. No formal exercise is required. Instead, you'll sneak more movement into your day by practicing "functional fitness" with our no-gym, no-equipment exercise plan. It's versatile, fun, and empowering. You'll love how it feels. You'll also take a 10-minute walk each evening after dinner that will ensure that your hearty meal doesn't go to your thighs and belly.

believing that your "dirty" organs are in need of Mr. Clean. Marketing people love the word "detox" because it sounds so proactive and healthy. You don't need detoxification, but your foods do.

The 7-Day Smoothie Diet is a plan that does the detoxification outside your body by cleaning up your food choices long before you open your mouth. By following this plan, you will replace highly processed snacks and meals full of added sugars and preservatives with whole foods, including nutritious smoothies made with whole foods.

You'll love the simplicity of this diet program. It works on auto-pilot: All you have to do is drink two delicious smoothies, one in the morning and one later on, and you will automatically reduce the number of calories you consume in one day, leading to sustainable weight loss. Smoothies can support weight loss in other ways besides reducing calories while boosting satiety: When you drink smoothies made with colorful vegetables and fruits, your body gets a huge influx of healthful plant compounds called flavonoids that make it harder to gain weight. A recent study in the *British Medical Journal* found that out of 124,000 people middle-aged or older, those who ate a flavonoid-rich diet had much more success maintaining their weight than those who didn't. Other research suggests the many ways smoothies can be one of the best weapons against weight gain.

The Healthy Body Benefits of the Plan

A rich and creamy smoothie is one of the best weapons against weight gain because it...

- **satisfies hunger by adding volume to your stomach, fiber- and protein-rich liquid volume that is digested more slowly compared to sugary, processed foods**
- is quick and easy to prepare, ideal for those times when you don't have time to make a snack or meal...like every morning. Eating a protein-rich breakfast is an effective way to lose weight. In fact, a recent study in the journal *Obesity Research* discovered that 78 percent of study participants who ate breakfast daily lost an average of 70 pounds and kept it off for six years. If you are one of those people who just can't eat a traditional breakfast, a smoothie may be a very palatable way to fill your empty belly and prevent mid-morning doughnut binging
- **satisfies your desire for the rich, creamy mouth-feel of a shake**
- is loaded with vitamins and minerals, when made right, that you might be missing in your diet
- **is an easy way to front-load your diet with more vegetables**
- is packed with satiating, muscle-growing protein. If you are not getting your recommended amount of protein, a smoothie is great way to get more. If you don't eat meat, you can use high-quality vegetable-based protein powders that ensure you get the protein you need
- **is one of the best ways to sneak more fiber into your diet to keep hunger at bay, support a healthful gut biome, and keep your bathroom habits regular and healthy**
- can act as the foundation of a diet and fitness plan to keep you lean and healthy for life.

Here's the nitty-gritty of the 7-Day Smoothie Diet program:

- Drink a rich, thick, satisfying smoothie in the morning as a meal replacement for breakfast.
- **Eat a generous lunch, featuring lean protein and vegetables.**
- Drink a smoothie in the aftenoon to clobber hunger until dinnertime.
- **Eat a dinner of vegetables, lean proteins, maybe a little high-fiber pasta, almost anything you wish, except breads, starchy vegetables, or highly processed foods. Stick to one serving. If still hungry, have some more non-starchy vegetables.**

That's the basic eating plan to effectively slash significant calories from your daily intake and set you on a solid path toward a leaner, healthier body. Think you can handle that for seven days? I do. In fact, I think you'll really enjoy the program. It'll inspire you to continue to take charge of your health and the shape of your body so you can enjoy an active life to the fullest for a very long time.

Jeff Csatari
Executive Editor,
Eat This, Not That! Books

CHAPTER 1

A Head Start to Success

THIS SEVEN-DAY PLAN can help anyone who wants to clean up his or her diet. But it's also specifically designed for people who want to experience quick weight-loss results and the continued motivation that comes from feeling better and looking leaner quickly.

In a nutshell, the 7-Day Smoothie Diet works by significantly reducing your calorie consumption without you feeling the reduction. In other words, you won't feel as if you are starving, the hallmark of other low-calorie diets. By satisfying your hunger strategically, you avoid cravings, overeating, and packing on pounds.

Are You Sensitive to Carbs?

If you have struggled with weight gain in the past, there's a good chance you may be "carb sensitive." People who are sensitive to carbohydrates experience an exaggerated physiological response to sugars and carbohydrates. They get intense cravings for starches and sweets, or a ravenous appetite that leads to overeating and results in easy fat storage.

Take the Carb Sensitivity Self-Test

Check mark each statement that applies to you.

__ I am overweight. (See the Height-Weight Chart on the next page: Do you weigh more than the weight listed for your height?)
__ I have a parent or sibling with type 2 diabetes.
__ I often crave sweets or starches (bread, pasta, etc.).
__ I tend to eat when I'm feeling stressed.
__ I tend to gain weight in my belly.
__ I often feel sleepy an hour after eating a high-carb snack or meal.
__ I crave breakfast breads or cereal first thing in the morning.
__ I feel I need a sweet after every meal.
__ When eating a high-carb snack, I have trouble limiting how much I eat.
__ I often still feel hungry after a meal.

Score Yourself:
Count the number of checkmarks.

1-3: You may be slightly carb sensitive.
4-6: You are probably moderately carb sensitive.
7-10: It's very likely that you are very sensitive to carbohydrates.

AT-RISK WEIGHT CHART

Height	Weight (lbs.)	Height	Weight (lbs.)
4' 10"	129	5' 7"	172
4' 11"	133	5' 8"	177
5' 0"	138	5' 9"	182
5' 1"	143	5' 10"	188
5' 2"	147	5' 11"	193
5' 3"	152	6' 0"	199
5' 4"	157	6' 1"	204
5' 5"	162	6' 2"	210
5' 6"	167	6' 3"	216
		6' 4"	221

* Adapted from the CDC National Diabetes Prevention Program.

Obviously, this self-quiz isn't a blood test. And we are not doctors. But your answers to this quick quiz can point you to a potential sensitivity to carbohydrates that you can begin to control using the advice, techniques, and, yes, the smoothie recipes in this book.

(If you are concerned about carb sensitivity or type 2 diabetes, we highly recommend you visit your doctor for a full health evaluation. Ask specifically for an HA1c blood test, a highly accurate measurement of blood sugar level.)

We can tell you're ready to rev up your blender. But first, here's an overview of what you can expect to experience by following this simple, seven-day plan:

- weight loss of seven to 10 pounds in seven days
- more energy, mental clarity, confidence, and feelings of being in control of life
- better blood sugar control and fewer cravings for sweets
- improved digestive health and regular bathroom habits
- better sleep
- smoother skin.

You'll start to feel stronger, fitter, and younger in about a week, and that's where the real, life-changing benefit kicks in: You'll feel so good, you'll want more of those feelings, which will motivate you to adopt the 7-Day Smoothie Diet lifestyle for life.

Ok, let's get going! While reading this book, we'd like you to begin preparing for the seven days ahead. Think of it as a warm-up. Don't worry, it won't take much time, but this head start to the seven-day plan will be well worth the effort. Two days of mind and kitchen preparation will help you learn to overcome emotional eating and literally follow your gut. You'll learn the truth about your eating habits so you can make them healthier. You'll purge from your home the highly processed foods that are causing you to overeat, and you'll stock up on the strategically nutritious groceries you'll need during the 7-Day Smoothie Diet. And you'll begin slashing significant calories from your daily consumption without even feeling the change.

START HERE

Prep Day 1

A big part of 7-Day Smoothie Diet success hinges upon doing something pretty simple: cutting out the sugary beverages that add considerable calories your daily total. We're going to ask you to start that today.

Think about this: The average American consumes 224 calories every day just from sodas, sweet tea, fruit juices, and other sugary drinks. Have you ever grabbed a 64-ounce fountain cola drink from a convenience store on a hot summer day? That cup contains about 700 sugary calories! Liquid calories don't fill you up, but they can make you fat. A 20-year study of 120,000 men and women published in the journal *Lancet* found that people who increased their consumption of sugary drinks by just one 12-ounce serving per day gained more weight—a pound every four years—compared to people who did not drink more.

So, to get ready to lose weight rapidly, let's stop drinking the sugar water, beginning with Prep Day 1.

Upon waking up, we want you to drink 16 ounces of water, cold or warm, with a squeeze of lemon added. This is a healthy ritual we want you to adopt for life. The practice signals your body to start the day, it adds no-calorie volume to your empty belly, and if warm, it should encourage you to poop—all good for a healthy digestive system. When you begin the 7-Day Smoothie Diet, you will drink another tall glass of water before lunch and one before dinner, which will help fill your belly so you consume fewer calories during those meals. A recent study published in the journal *Obesity* found that drinking that much water before every meal helped people lose twice as much weight as people who didn't drink water, an average of 5.3 pounds over 12 weeks without doing anything else to lose weight. So drink to your health and gain the added weight loss boost.

If you normally drink hot tea or coffee in the morning, you can still have it, but only after drinking your morning lemon water. Cut the amount of milk or creamer and sugar in half, if you use any. It is important to begin to recognize how much sugar you consume daily purely from sweetened beverages and how little you actually need it.

Limit yourself to just one more cup of coffee or tea the rest of the day, this time black and unsweetened. Do not drink soda, juices, or alcohol today. Might as well get in the habit; you will drink only water, unsweetened iced tea, unsweetened coffee or hot tea, or calorie-free sparkling water during the 7-Day Smoothie Diet. Except, of course, smoothies!

How to Eat on Prep Day 1

Eat as you normally do. There are no recommended food changes today other than the avoidance of sweetened beverages. Record everything you eat and drink and how much, as best as you can estimate. Use a notebook or the sample tracker on the next page.

Record your mood and hunger levels, as well as how you feel about missing those sweetened drinks. And write down your bedtime and wakeup time.

PREP DAY 1 FOOD TRACKER

Date ____________________ Awoke at __________ a.m.

BREAKFAST: ______________________________

Beverage: ______________________________

Calories: ______________________________

SNACK (only if eaten): ______________________________

Beverage: ______________________________

Calories: ______________________________

LUNCH: ______________________________

Beverage: ______________________________

Calories: ______________________________

SNACK (only if eaten): ______________________________

Beverage: ______________________________

Calories: ______________________________

DINNER: ______________________________

Beverage: ______________________________

Calories: ______________________________

DESSERT (if eaten): ______________________________

Beverage: ______________________________

Calories: ______________________________

SNACK (only if eaten): ______________________________

Beverage: ______________________________

Calories: ______________________________

TOTAL CALORIES: ______________________________

BEDTIME: ______________________________

HUNGER LEVEL: 1 2 3 4 5

(5 = very hungry; 3 = moderately hungry; 1 = not hungry)

MOOD LEVEL: 1 2 3 4 5

(5 = irritable or depressed; 4 = meh; 1 = calm and happy

PHYSICAL ACTIVITY: ______________________________

Prep Day 2

Upon waking up, drink 16 ounces of cold or warm lemon water. Today, drink your hot tea and coffee black, this time without any sugar.

While having your coffee, review yesterday's Food Tracker. What did you eat? How much of what you ate was starchy carbohydrates or sweets? How many vegetables did you eat? How about whole grains? Get a sense of how much protein you ate in relation to the starches. How many total calories did you consume? The point of this exercise is not to learn to count calories but rather to get a better understanding of what kinds of foods you are eating most, how much food you are consuming, when, where, and why. The more you know about your eating style, the easier it will be to recognize when you are leaning toward unhealthy choices and the easier it will be to make adjustments.

Is your tracker painting a picture of overeating? Are you finding you are mindlessly munching? Can you tell from your tracker whether you are eating as the result of stress or high emotion? Keeping a food log is an eye-opening exercise. Even when you record your meals for only a day or two, you can learn a lot about your eating habits and the types of foods you gravitate toward. It can surprise you or simply confirm your intuition about how you eat. Regularly logging your meals either on paper or online can be another weapon in your arsenal of weight-loss tools. One study of nearly 1,700 people from Kaiser Permanente's Center for Health Research found that keeping a food log can double a person's weight loss.

Keep a food log today and then for the full 7-Day Smoothie Diet challenge to stay on track. For Prep Day 2, we are going to adjust the rules a bit.

For Prep Day 2, we'd like you to skip breakfast—no smoothies, no eggs or doughnuts, nothing. Why? We want you to recognize how hungry you feel at around 10 a.m. You'll probably be famished. Record your hunger level and mood. Be mindful of your cravings. How does skipping breakfast affect your choice of mid-morning snack? Have whatever you want for a snack, but record what you choose and how it satisfies you before lunch. Do you end up eating a larger snack than usual?

If you are still hungry after your snack, have a tall glass of water, wait 10 minutes, and record your hunger again. Lunch will be here soon enough!

Continue to avoid beverages with added sugars. Record your mood and hunger levels, as well as how you feel about missing those sweetened drinks. Is there any change?

Try to make it to lunchtime before eating again.

Lunch

For lunch between noon and 1:30 p.m., have one of the following:

* **A large green salad** containing protein—chicken breast,

sliced hard-boiled eggs, tuna, and/or beans or legumes. You can have any dressing you would like, but be mindful of how much you pour on your salad. Remember, it's salad, not soup!

OR

A sandwich on whole-wheat bread. Filling can be turkey deli meat, chicken breast, roast beef, tuna salad with light mayonnaise, or veggies (lettuce, hummus, avocado, sliced bell peppers, sprouts, etc.). Have some baby carrots or celery with spicy red pepper hummus for dipping, if you'd like.

3 P.M.

If you are hungry, you may have a handful of raw almonds or a cheese stick. If you are not hungry, avoid having a snack.

Record your mood and hunger levels just before dinner.

Dinner

Pour yourself a large glass of ice water (16 ounces) to have with your meal. Eat what you normally do. But don't have seconds. Try to start off with a broth-based soup, like minestrone or chicken noodle, or a salad to fill you up. No seconds on the main course, but have as many vegetables as you'd like. Don't drink any alcohol with dinner or after.

Do not have dessert or anything to eat after 7 p.m.

Record your mood and hunger levels. At the end of the day, review your Food Log. How did it differ from Day 1? Did you learn anything new about your eating habits or how you feel?

PREP DAY 2 FOOD TRACKER

Date ____________________ Awoke at ________________ a.m.

16 ounces of lemon water.

BREAKFAST: Skip breakfast today. We want you to recognize feelings of hunger at midmorning and how it impacts your snack choices. You may have a cup of black coffee or tea without sugar or milk.

Beverage: ____________________

SNACK (only if eaten): ____________________

Beverage: ____________________

Calories: ____________________

Record your hunger and mood levels. ____________________

LUNCH: ____________________

Beverage: ____________________

Calories: ____________________

SNACK (only if eaten): ____________________

Beverage: ____________________

DINNER: ____________________

Beverage (no alcohol): ____________________

Calories: ____________________

Be mindful: Did skipping breakfast this morning affect your dinner choice and how many calories you consumed?

TOTAL CALORIES: ____________________

BEDTIME: ____________________

HUNGER LEVEL: 1 2 3 4 5

(5 = very hungry; 3 = moderately hungry; 1 = not hungry)

MOOD LEVEL: 1 2 3 4 5

(5 = irritable or depressed; 4 = meh; 1 = calm and happy

PHYSICAL ACTIVITY: ______________________

Prep Day 2 Activity: The Kitchen Cleanse

There's a ton of sugar-heavy, processed junk food lurking in your refrigerator and pantry. It's not doing you any favors. Toss it out or at least get it out of sight during the 7-Day Smoothie Diet. You don't need the temptation to snack on this stuff when you are trying to change your eating habits and lose some weight.

"Get a trash bag, go through your fridge and pantry, and throw out all of the expired food and junk food you know is not good for your health! If it's not in the house, you won't eat it," says nutritionist Lisa DeFazio, MS, RDN.

What to purge and why: See the "Toss It Hit List" on page 18 for a checklist of stuff to get rid of. You may come across some food items that you think are good to have on hand because they seem like traditionally healthy choices. Let's take a moment to learn the real deal about foods with this kind of "health halo."

Cold cereals. Most—even the ones that seem healthy—are carb-laden, sweet, and highly processed. They are not the breakfast of champions by any means. Toss 'em. You're going to be starting your day—at least for the first week of our program—with a rich, thick, protein-based smoothie. After seven days, you may opt out of the breakfast smoothie and replace it with a breakfast of lean protein, like eggs, the best way to ensure that you'll stay energized and full into early afternoon.

Cream-based soups. As you'll learn in this book, having a soup appetizer is an effective way to reduce the overall calories in a meal. You fill your belly with the soothing hot liquid and end up eating less for the main course. But this only works if that soup you're eating is broth-based, which is typically lower in calories than cream-based soups. Creamy soups are usually loaded with empty calories and often have concerning fillers like hydrolyzed proteins, food dyes, and corn syrup, warns Dr. Taz Bhatia, an integrative health expert. Choose a broth-based soup to start your meal. You get bonus points if it contains protein, too. A bowl of black bean soup, for example, is an ideal precursor to a vegetable salad. You get volume, fiber, and protein, all of which add up to a satisfied belly.

Deli meats, even turkey breast. "While the link between meat and chronic disease is fairly tenuous, the connection between salt-, sugar-, and chemical-laden processed meats and chronic disease risk is strong and consistent," says David L. Katz, MD, MPH, president of the American College of Lifestyle Medicine and an advisor to *Eat This, Not That!* "If you eat meat, it should be pure—like you want your own muscles to be. If you eat the highly processed, adulterated meats they may pay it forward to the meat on your own bones."

Diet sodas. They contain phosphorus, which binds to calcium and increases calcium loss, which is terrible for bone health, according to orthopedic surgeons. And they are made with artificial sweeteners that have potentially dangerous effects on the brain and metabolism.

Dried fruit. The fructose gets more concentrated when fruit is dried out, making it more potent in smaller doses. Also, many companies top their dried fruits with additional sugars and coating, making it even more sugary.

Energy bars, including protein bars. They're often high in excess calories, sugar, fat, and carbohydrates and are filled with an endless list of chemicals. Frequently we'll see people treating protein bars as "snacks" when they really should be considered a meal replacement.

Flavored instant oatmeal. Although instant oats are a timesaving way to get a fiber-rich breakfast, many are laden with chemical additives, sugars, and inflammatory oils. Check the ingredients lists and sugar content on the labels.

Granola. Granola is one of the leading health food impostors. One cup of granola has nearly 600 calories, 30 grams of fat, and 24 grams of sugar. That's the equivalent of two slices of cheesecake.

Hazelnut spreads like Nutella. These spreads seem healthy to many people because they contain a nut, and nuts are supposed to be good for you. But check the ingredients label on these spreads, and you'll see that they are made primarily of sugar (often more than 20 grams) and palm oil, with almost no actual nuts involved.

Orange juice. When you take an orange and transform it into juice, you take away its fiber—one of the major benefits of consuming whole fruits and vegetables. (Same goes for apples, grapes—any fruit.) What you wind up with is a drink that's so concentrated with sweetness, it can have as much sugar as a soda. Instead eat whole fruits, especially dark ones like raspberries, strawberries, and blueberries, which are packed with polyphenols, powerful natural chemicals that can actually stop fat from forming.

Packaged baked goods marketed as "low-fat." To make up for the lack of fat, food manufacturers pack these extensively processed foods with chemicals that try to reproduce the consistency and flavor of the full-fat originals. Keep them out of your house.

Pre-packaged microwave popcorn. Popcorn is filled with healthy fiber and grains, but only if you get the air-popped versions. Many pre-packaged microwave popcorns contain heart-harming trans fats and the dangerous butter-flavor additive diacetyl, an ingredient shown to harm the brain.

Rice cakes. These are an old-school diet staple. But the simple carbohydrates rank notoriously high on the glycemic index (GI)—a measure of how quickly blood sugar rises in response to food on a scale of 1 to 100 (rice cakes come in at 82). High GI foods provide a rush of energy but can leave you hungry within a few hours. Researchers at the New Balance Foundation Obesity Prevention Center found high-GI snacks caused excessive hunger and increased activity in the craving and reward area of the brain—the perfect storm for overeating and weight gain.

Now, if you can't bear to toss a newly bought pack of rice cakes, put it back in your pantry. Just stay away from it during your 7-Day Smoothie Diet and then do this: Instead of eating a two-cake serving, take one cake and top it with a generous swipe of almond butter for a cravings buster snack. The combo of carbs, fiber, fats, and protein (complete protein with all nine essential amino acids) will keep you fuller longer.

Spinach wraps. While the leafy green is packed full of vital nutrients our bodies need each day, those wraps made with spinach tortillas have so little of the green stuff that they won't do your body any good. The wraps are typically made with the same refined ingredients of other tortillas—like enriched white flour—and green food coloring that gives them the healthy green look. Sneaky!

Veggie chips. Veggie chips are not vegetables. Far from them. The way the vegetables are processed into chips in manufacturing plants means you're getting a ton of sodium (and maybe even sugar) without all of the nutrients. Baked chips are also touted as a healthier alternative to regular potato chips, since those crunchy snacks are typically fried in oil. While it is true that baked chips are lower in fat, they're typically processed with a ton of added sodium and sugar to improve flavor. Crunch into some raw carrots or celery sticks instead.

Sweetened or fruit-added yogurt. Yogurt is a wonderful food; the probiotics found in it are great for your gut, plus it's loaded with protein. But the health benefits are wiped out when you eat the flavored versions sold at stores. The reason: They're loaded with sugar—sometimes 20 grams or more for just a few ounces of yogurt. Keep yogurt healthy by looking for low-sugar versions (ideally less than 8 grams), and add a bit of honey or berries for taste.

Those are the main healthy-food impostors you probably have in your home right now. Do a clean sweep of them so you will not be tempted or misled by them during the 7-Day Smoothie Diet.

COUNTER TEMPTATION

Eat clean by keeping a tidy kitchen.

Want to make it easier to avoid mindless eating? Tidy up your kitchen. If your kitchen counter is cluttered and disorganized, you'll likely overeat there, research suggests. In one study, people who saw snack foods on cluttered kitchen counters ate 44 percent more food than people who saw the same snacks on very neat countertops.

Keep food out of sight and you'll be less likely to be tempted, according to studies at Cornell University's Food and Brand Lab. In one study, researchers found that people who had chips or cookies visible on their kitchen counters weighed about 10 pounds more than people with bare kitchen counters. Breakfast cereal boxes left on kitchen counters led to greater consumption and weight gain, too. Study participants who kept cereal in plain view weighed about 21 pounds more than people who kept their cereals out of sight in a cabinet.

"Simply the presence of food is a really powerful cue to eat," says Brian Wansink, director of the Cornell lab and author of *Slim by Design: Mindless Eating Solutions for Everyday Life.*

TOSS IT HIT LIST

PANTRY

- Candy
- Cookies
- Brown sugar
- Potato chips
- Pretzels
- Dried fruit
- Crackers
- Pasta (unless it's made from whole wheat, chickpea, or lentil flour)
- Rice
- Sugary breakfast cereals
- Cakes
- White bread

REFRIGERATOR

- Fruit drinks, juices, and sodas
- Applesauce
- Jelly and jam
- Ketchup
- Barbecue sauce and other bottled sauces and salsas

FREEZER

- Ice cream
- Frozen waffles
- Cakes
- Muffins
- Dough
- Frozen breads
- Bagels
- Frozen pizza

CHAPTER

2

Rule #1
Drink Two Satisfying Shakes

THIS IS THE backbone of the 7-Day Smoothie Diet plan: You'll drink one rich smoothie for breakfast each morning and one lighter smoothie in the afternoon as a between-lunch-and-dinner snack. Simple. Quick. Delicious. Nutritious.

It's important to note the difference between blending shake-like smoothies and juicing. When you juice, the pulp, where all that good-for-you fiber is found, is discarded. Smoothies are blended with whole foods, and the fiber stays suspended in the liquid so you get it into your gut. Why is that important? Because fiber slows the digestion of food and puts the brakes on sugars so they don't enter the bloodstream too quickly; when sugars enter the bloodstream too rapidly, they cause spikes that quickly dip and trigger cravings. Smoothies are thicker than juices, keeping you feeling full much longer. Juice quickly empties from the stomach, causing you to become hungry again not long after drinking. By blending your smoothies with the right ingredients—proteins, fiber-rich carbohydrates, and healthy fats—you create a drink that acts like a hearty meal, one that balances your blood sugar and helps with weight control.

Now you might be wondering, why not just eat breakfast instead of drink a smoothie?

Good question. But before we answer, we have one for you: Do you eat a high-protein, fiber-rich breakfast every day? Do you have, say, a vegetable omelet with Canadian bacon and a piece of whole-grain toast or maybe plain Greek yogurt with fresh berries and crushed walnuts?

Most American's don't. If they eat a morning meal, typically it's something quick and often packaged: a bowl of cereal, a bagel, a granola bar, or, worse, a doughnut or croissant. Let's look at some of those options: Boxed cereal, even if it boasts "made with whole grains" on the front, may contain upward of 18 grams of sugar. Even oatmeal can mislead you. For example: McDonald's Fruit & Maple Oatmeal sounds like a better choice than a doughnut, but it still contains 32 grams of sugar. That's almost as much as you'd find in two Hostess Ding Dongs. How about a bagel and cream cheese? Filling, right? Well, that's because today's typical bagel is supersized at four inches in diameter. One is actually the equivalent of four servings. Plus, it's made with white flour, the kind that elevates blood sugar very quickly.

In the hustle and bustle of the morning's rush out the door, we often don't have time to make a hot, nutritious breakfast, so we grab and go. And what we grab is typically packaged and highly processed or full of fast-burning, low-fiber carbohydrates and little protein.

Many people skip the morning meal completely—due to lack of time or because they don't like to eat in the morning. At work several hours later they often become ravenous, raiding the vending machine or the box of doughnuts a coworker brought in to celebrate Chuck in accounting's birthday.

Eating after the nighttime fast is important because your body needs good fuel to work optimally. That's especially true of your brain, which is powered by glucose you get from food. But eating in the morning can also enhance your weight loss by revving up your metabolism, which starts your calorie burn. A few years back, Virginia Commonwealth University researchers conducted a study involving one group of dieters who started each day with a protein-rich breakfast and another group who consumed only a quarter of the first group's protein. The big breakfast eaters lost more weight and found it easier to adhere to their diets despite the fact that each group ate roughly the same number of calories for the morning meal. Many other studies point toward the weight-loss benefits of eating breakfast. One analysis of successful dieters found that 78 percent of them eat breakfast every day. And a landmark University of Massachusetts study determined that people who usually skip breakfast are 450 percent more likely to end up obese.

Rise and Dine

Eat big in the a.m. to lose weight.

Eating a high-energy breakfast helped obese diabetics lose weight and reduce their need for insulin, according to a new study from Tel Aviv University presented at the Endocrine Society. While the study involved people with type 2 diabetes, the takeaway—that when you eat is just as important as what you eat—may be useful to anyone trying to control hunger and lose weight. In the study, men and women were randomly assigned to one of two weight-loss diets containing equal amounts of calories. One group ate three meals a day: a large breakfast and a smaller lunch and dinner. The other group ate six small meals, including snacks, spaced throughout the day. Six small meals are typically recommended for diabetics to keep blood sugar levels stable and reduce cravings. But this study demonstrated that carbohydrate cravings and hunger decreased significantly in the big-breakfast group, but not the six-meals group. What's more, blood sugar levels decreased signicantly in only the big-breakfast eaters, and they lost 11 pounds in three months compared to only three pounds for the other dieters.

The Breakfast Smoothie

For the next seven days, we'd like you to drink a breakfast smoothie within a half hour of having your wake-up lemon water. Starting the day off with a smoothie with a roughly even portion of high-quality protein and good carbohydrates will pull your body out of its overnight fasting state by giving you quick energy. The fiber, fat, and protein inside will ensure that your first meal sticks with you for hours.

If you normally eat some kind of breakfast, you'll find that our recommended smoothies are filling, tasty, and satisfying. If you don't normally eat breakfast, this seven-day plan will be a good jumpstart for the practice. We think you'll quickly see that filling your stomach with the right foods improves your alertness, reduces cravings for sweets, and keeps your belly from grumbling in late morning. You'll also likely notice that you won't eat as much food the rest of the day.

Drinking a protein-rich smoothie as a breakfast meal replacement for a carbohydrate-heavy or fat-rich breakfast can help you consume fewer calories at lunchtime, according to a study in the *European Journal of Clinical Nutrition*.

While research is ongoing, new studies suggest that timing of calorie consumption may play a significant roll in weight loss. In one experiment at the University of Alabama in Birmingham, scientists placed a small group of people on two different eating plans. In the first, the participants started eating at 8 a.m. and had their last meal at 2 p.m. In the second plan, they spread out their meals between 8 a.m. and 8 p.m. While the subjects consumed the same number of calories on both schedules, researchers found that they burned 6 percent more fat when they ate most of their calories earlier in the day. What's more, the participants reported feeling less hungry throughout the day, even though their window of eating was compressed.

Cereal Killer

Have you ever measured the flakes you shake into your bowl?

Here's an eye-opening exercise for all you boxed cereal eaters out there. Grab what you think is your healthiest cold cereal in your pantry. Maybe it's cornflakes, maybe it's muesli or granola or something touted for its nuts and fiber. Doesn't matter. Dump it in a bowl as you normally do. But don't add milk. Instead, look at the recommended serving size on the nutrition facts panel. Now grab a set of small measuring cups—¼ cup to 1 cup. Use the serving cup that matches the serving size, and use it to start shoveling the cereal back into the box. Count how many servings you put back. That's how many you typically eat. Now have a good look at how tiny that single serving really is. Puny. That's why we're asking you to dump your cold cereal habit and drink a substantial morning smoothie that will stick with you until lunch.

We're not going to ask you to stop eating at two p.m. Hey, we love eating dinner, too! But we do strongly believe that eating more of the right calories in the morning helps keep blood sugar—and hunger—more stable throughout the day, which is critical for losing weight.

Do this: Choose one of the Breakfast Smoothies or a Breakfast Smoothie Bowl from Chapter 4 for each morning meal. These smoothies are designed to be higher in calories and high-quality carbohydrates than the afternoon smoothies. In the morning, after a night of nothing in your belly, you need something substantial, with protein and good carbs, to fuel your body and brain. Many of these smoothies also contain healthy fats like nuts or olive oil and coconut oil. Fats provide a rich and satisfying mouth-feel that you'll enjoy and they will satisfy your belly's craving for something substantial. Like protein and fiber, fats take lon-

ger to digest than simple carbohydrates (sugars) do, keeping you feeling fuller longer. Drinking one of these smoothies around 7:30 or 8 a.m. should keep you energized and full until just before lunchtime. If you find yourself getting hungry or craving carbs before lunch, drink a glass of ice water or use one of the many Cravings Crushers techniques found in Chapter 6 to get you over the hump.

Here are two of our favorite smoothie recipes for a morning meal: First is a "good-fat" smoothie. Second is a smoothie bowl, for those who prefer to use a spoon.

Chocolate Peanut Butter Power Smoothie

1 banana, sliced
⅓ cup tofu, cut into cubes
½ cup spinach or kale, washed and dried
1 cup milk or almond milk
¼ cup Greek yogurt
1 Tbsp. smooth peanut butter
2 tsp. local honey
2 tsp. cocoa powder
1 tsp. chia seeds

- Add the banana slices, tofu cubes, and spinach or kale to a blender. Top with ½ cup of almond milk and Greek yogurt. Blend on high until smooth.
- Add the peanut butter, honey, cocoa powder, chia seeds, and the rest of the milk. Blend again until smooth.

Makes two servings.
Per serving: 301 calories, 9 g fat, 45 g carbohydrates, 5 g fiber, 19 g protein
(For more breakfast smoothie recipes, see page 49 and 131.)

Toppings Stopper: A quick note about those lovin' spoonfuls of tasty treats that you sprinkle on top of smoothies and smoothie bowls: Please be mindful of your toppings choices. Avoid those high in sugar, like most dried fruits and candies like M&Ms. (Yes, we've seen people dump M&Ms and crushed Health Bars on their smoothie bowls!) Some much healthier toppings include:

BERRIES—High in antioxidants and fiber

ROLLED OATS—Contain a fiber called beta-glucan that regulates blood sugar and slashes cholesterol

NUTS AND SEEDS (Almonds, pistachios, walnuts, sunflower seeds, flaxseeds, and pumpkin seeds)—Many are rich in heart-healthy plant-based omega-3 fats, vitamin E, and other nutrients

---

The Blueberry Cobbler Bowl

1 cup frozen blueberries
½ cup unsweetened almond milk
1½ scoops protein powder
2 Tbsp. almond butter
1 tsp. vanilla extract

THE TOPPINGS:

½ cup fresh blueberries or strawberries
¼ cup vanilla granola
2 Tbsp. sliced almonds
2 tsp. hemp seeds
1 tsp. cinnamon

- Blend the first five ingredients until smooth. Pour into bowls and top with the toppings.

Makes 2 servings.

Per serving: 372 calories, 16 g fat, 32 g carbohydrates, 7 g fiber, 25 g protein

(For more smoothie bowl recipes, see page 53 and 139.)

The Afternoon Smoothie

Have you ever noticed that when you are really busy at work or at home, you can power through the day and forget to break for lunch? What happens when you finish the job or things slow down later in the day? Right, your belly reminds you, "Hey, you forgot to feed me." Suddenly, eating becomes urgent and you start hunting for the quick and tasty—and high in calories. That's your survival instinct kicking into high gear: Your brain instinctively tells you to seek high-fat, high-calorie sustenance just in case you have to go for a length of time without eating again.

That's why we want you to have a filling, protein-rich lunch, and never skip it. The next chapter will detail the principle behind eating an extra-filling meal, but the purpose of the afternoon smoothie is similar: avoiding feelings of ravenous hunger that override rational, mindful eating habits. Each day at about 3 p.m. or when you start to feel emptiness in your belly, drink a delicious smoothie from the list of recipes on page 54. These smoothies are lower in calories than your morning smoothies because they aren't supposed to be meal replacements. Instead, they are snack replacements, designed to be lower in calories than that bag of pretzels, scoop of ice cream, or package of Twinkies you're snacking on in the afternoon. Low in sugar, they will help you avoid the 4 p.m. sleepies that come from eating heavier carb-laden snacks late in the day. Weighing in at around 300 calories or less, these smoothies will give you a burst of energy and fill your belly to tide you over until dinnertime. By having something in the late afternoon, you will fend off the intense, urgent feelings that make you say, "I'm starving. I could eat a rhinoceros, even though I'm a vegetarian."

Below are two examples of perfect afternoon smoothie recipes. The first contains no raw fruits or vegetables for practical reasons: If you work in an office or at a jobsite, you probably don't have access to a high-powered blender required to pulverize produce. So, simplify things by using just protein powder and some almond milk. You can use a plastic tumbler with a secure top and one of those metal or plastic shaker balls inside to whip the contents into a frothy consistency. Even better, try the nonelectric portable "blender" called the Revablend. It features a rubber base that you roll back and forth on a flat surface at a 30-degree angle to spin metal blender blades inside. Five or six revs pulverizes those globules of unblended protein powder you sometimes get with those shaker ball containers. The Revablend blades can even handle a ripe banana.

Easy Chocolate Protein Snack

10 oz. unsweetened almond milk or water
2 scoops chocolate protein powder such as Orgain Organic Meal Creamy Chocolate Fudge

Makes 1 serving.

Per serving: 220 calories, 5 g fat, 24 g carbohydrates, 8 g fiber, 20 g protein

The Coffee Break Smoothie

½ cup brewed coffee
(use decaf if caffeine late in the day affects your sleep)
½ large banana, cut into chunks
½ cup plain Greek yogurt
½ Tbsp. ground flaxseed
1 tsp. local honey
¼ tsp. cinnamon
¼ tsp. grated nutmeg (optional)

Makes 1 serving.

Per serving: 135 calories, 1.3 g fat, 21 g carbohydrates, 2.4 g fiber, 9 g protein

(For more afternoon smoothie recipes, see page 54.)

The 7-Day Smoothie Diet features a plan to move your body more throughout the day without having to go to a gym or a use traditional strength-training equipment or aerobic machines. But if you already work out in a gym and do strenuous workouts in the afternoon, you may want to drink a protein-rich post-workout smoothie that contains more calories than this or the other suggested afternoon smoothies you'll find on page 54. For an after-exercise smoothie, you can choose one of the breakfast smoothies in Chapter 4.

If it's too inconvenient to blend a protein shake at work, consider making a batch at home and bringing a tumbler full to work in a small cooler. Or buy one of the premixed protein shakes in cardboard or plastic bottles from the grocery or health food store. They can be pricey. Some are loaded with sugars, calories, and chemical additives (see Calorie Bombs, page 31) and should be avoided. If you do some detective work, you can find some grab-and-go protein shakes that can easily serve as your afternoon smoothie. Hunt for premade shakes with no artificial sweeteners, high-fructose corn syrup, or hydrogenated oils. Here are a few that good ones that have at least 12 grams of high-quality proteins and deliver the right blend of amino acids required to build and repair muscle tissues. Unless otherwise mentioned, these products are sweetened with either stevia or stevia and monk fruit extract, two of *Eat This, Not That!*'s favorite non-nutritive sweeteners.

Skinnygirl Protein Shake

Per 11.5 oz. bottle: 80 calories, 1.5 g fat (1 g saturated fat), 350 mg sodium, 5 g carbohydrates, 3 g fiber, 12 g protein

---

Orgain Organic Nutritional Shake

Per 11 oz. bottle: 255 calories, 7 g fat (1 g saturated fat), 260 mg sodium, 32 g carbohydrates, 2 g fiber, 16 g protein

---

Orgain Vegan Nutritional Shake

Per 11 oz. bottle: 220 calories, 6 g fat (1 g saturated fat), 160–185 mg sodium, 25 g carbohydrates, 2 g fiber, 16 g protein

---

FitPro Go!

Per 14 oz. bottle, vanilla: 200 calories, 2.5 g fat (1 g saturated fat), 400 mg sodium, 10 g carbohydrates, 2 g fiber, 35 g protein

---

Iconic Lean Protein Shake

Per 11.5 oz. bottle: 130 calories, 2 g fat (0 g saturated fat), 8 g carbohydrates, 4 g fiber, 20 g protein

Stonyfield OP Organic Protein Vanilla Smoothie

Per 11 oz. bottle: 190 calories, 2 g fat (1.5 g saturated fat), 170 mg sodium, 26 g carbohydrates, 1 g fiber, 15 g protein

Muscle Milk Organic Non Dairy Protein Shake

Per 12 oz. bottle: 170 calories, 4 g fat (1 g saturated fat), 180 mg sodium, 14 g carbohydrates, 0 g fiber, 20 g protein

Calorie Bombs

Avoid most bottled smoothies.

Sure, a store-bought fruit smoothie is ultra-convenient and sounds like a virtuous choice for an afternoon pick-me-up, but most of these are loaded with shocking amounts of sugar and calories. Many are blended with high-calorie dairy bases and cheap sweeteners that make them more dessert-like than diet-friendly. For example, a small Baskin Robbins Mango Banana Smoothie packs 440 calories, nearly a third of what the average woman on a 1,500-calorie weight loss diet needs in an entire day. Not to mention 96 grams of sugar—that's more than you'll find in seven scoops of the chain's Rainbow Sherbet. Adding insult to injury, banana doesn't even appear on the ingredients list. Convenience store bottled smoothies can be ridiculously high in sugars and calories, too. For example, Naked Protein & Greens by Naked contains 59 grams of sugar and 400 calories in a 15.2-ounce bottle. A bottle of Odwalla Original Super Protein carries 350 calories and 56 grams of sugar. The World Health Organization recommends that we eat no more than 25 grams of sugar per day for optimal health, while the USDA recommends that we eat no more than 50 grams.

CHAPTER

3

Protein Powder Buyer's Guide

THE SHEER NUMBER of protein powders available online and on store shelves will make your head spin like the blades of a blender set on puree. They are not all created equal. Some are gritty, chalky, and don't blend well with other ingredients, while others are packed with sugar and artificial ingredients.

Choosing the wrong protein powder can actually derail your effort to lose weight. So we're going to make it easy for you. The protein powders on these pages are the ones we at *Eat This, Not That!* dump into our blenders along with our favorite produce and nut milk.

You can't go wrong with these. Still, you have a choice to make. There are two main categories of protein mixes for smoothies: animal-based protein supplements and plant-based protein powders. The former are made from eggs, whey, or casein protein. The vegan proteins are made from pea, hemp, rice, and soy proteins. Both are good for weight loss. If you are vegan, the choice is obvious. But even those who do eat meat may prefer plant-based proteins because they're lactose-free and usually lower in sugar, so they do a better job of fighting bloat and inflammation. Read through the descriptions and try a few different powders and flavors. You can often find single-serving pouches that make it easy to sample many different styles. Regardless of which type you choose, the best protein powders will provide at least 15 grams of protein per serving.

Plant-Based Proteins

Look for pea, hemp, soy, or rice powders, ideally in blends. Because many single-plant-based varieties aren't complete proteins, consuming a blended plant-protein powder (like one that contains both pea and rice, along with a variety of sprouts) will ensure you're getting more amino acids and thus the most bang for your supplement buck.

Sunwarrior Warrior Blend Raw Protein Powder

Protein source: Pea, hemp, cranberry protein, and brown rice
Protein payoff: 19 grams per serving
A great raw protein option, this GMO-free powder derives its muscle-building power from raw organic pea, cranberry, and hemp seed protein—it's even tasty enough to take on its own! What's more, there are no sugars, gluten, or artificial sweeteners to cause a metabolism-confusing midday crash.

This blend is also good for a pre-workout smoothie because its branched-chain amino acids can help shuttle energy directly to your muscles.

$44.99 ($1.12 per serving)

Vega One All-In-One Nutritional Shake

Protein source: Pea protein and hemp protein

Protein payoff: 20 grams per serving

Loaded with six servings of greens, probiotics, antioxidants and 50 percent of your daily intake of food-based vitamins and minerals, this super-clean option is difficult to turn down. With tasty flavors like vanilla chai and berry, adding water alone is enough to create a tasty shake you'll enjoy sipping. If you have more time, combine a scoop—which doles out 20 grams of protein—with unsweetened milk alternatives and a frozen banana for an irresistible milk shake–like creation. Created by a former Ironman triathlete, this balanced protein also tastes great in homemade protein muffins.

$49 ($2.45 per serving)

Garden of Life Raw Protein

Protein source: Organic sprouted protein blend (brown rice, amaranth, quinoa, and millet)

Protein payoff: 22 grams per serving

This complete protein showcases 13 raw and organic sprouts, with 22 grams of protein per serving, all the essential amino acids your body needs, plus tea and cinnamon extract. Just make sure you whip up a smoothie using a healthy fat like nut butter or avocado. Makers of this powder load it with fat-soluble vitamins A, D, E, and K, which can only be fully absorbed by your body when paired with a healthy fat. Their original unflavored powder works in any post-workout shake, but we're suckers for slimming, satisfying chocolate versions.

When you're looking for an option with rice, make sure the brand uses sprouted brown rice (like Garden of Life does), not just "rice protein." Sprouting the rice reduces the amount of carbs and increases the amount of protein, which lowers the glycemic effect (minimizing blood sugar spikes) and increases the nutritional profile. Plus, when rice protein is sprouted, it changes in genetic makeup to make its nutrients more bioavailable to the body, according to the Food and Agriculture Organization of the UN.

$31.25 ($1.56 per serving)

Nutiva Organic Hemp Protein

Protein source: Hemp

Protein payoff: 15 g per serving

Hemp protein is derived from the hemp plant, offering a substantial amount of fiber (here, 8 grams) that's easy to digest. On top of 15 grams of complete protein per serving, hemp also boasts heart-healthy doses of anti-inflammatory omega-3s. This option is an ideal mix-in for oatmeal or smoothies; the fiber will make you feel fuller longer, and it contains eight essential amino acids to build muscle.

$10.73 ($0.72 per serving)

Aloha Superfood Protein

Protein source: Hemp, pumpkin seeds, and peas
Protein payoff: 18 grams per serving
Milk the benefits of this tasty, plant-based protein powder by slipping it into one of your quick smoothies or shakes. The organic, vegan powder is made with hemp seeds, pumpkin seeds, and peas for an impressive punch of 18 grams of protein per serving—with no chemicals or artificial fillers. And while it may be gluten-free, soy-free, and dairy-free, it's certainly rich in flavor. When you try this in a shake recipe that is originally dairy-based, you'd swear it was the real thing from its rich texture and flavor. Try their wild harvested vanilla or fair trade organic cacao powder swirled into a quick shake with half a frozen banana for an ice cream–like texture and a tablespoon of nut butter for satiating healthy fats and some extra protein.
$28.49 ($1.86 per serving)

Amazing Grass Protein Superfood, Chocolate Peanut Butter

Protein Source: Organic pea protein, organic hemp protein, organic chia, organic quinoa
Protein payoff: 21 g per serving
This may not be the best tasting powder on the list, but it certainly is up there with the best for you. This superfood blend packs 21 grams of complete protein as well as two servings of organic fruits and vegetables. The company strives to use non-GMO, kosher, vegan, and gluten-free ingredients only, making their powders as raw as possible.
$45.14 ($2.50 per serving)

Orgain Organic Protein, Sweet Vanilla Bean

Protein Source: Organic pea protein, organic brown rice protein, organic chia seed, organic hemp protein

Protein payoff: 24 g per serving

This protein powder is made from some of the highest quality certified organic plant proteins. It is made with no hormones, no antibiotics, and no pesticides or herbicide residues. The company also eliminates any artificial colors, flavors, or preservatives. And better yet, all ingredients are sourced right in the USA. This powder is loaded with 24 grams of organic protein, 5 grams of belly-filling fiber, and a complete amino acid profile. The texture of this powder is as smooth as pancake batter — and it smells just like it! The flavor, however, is quite strong and sweet, almost too sweet for us, but definitely worth a shot for readers who love their dessert.

$25.49 ($1.27 per serving)

Sunwarrior Classic Protein

Protein Source: Raw whole grain brown rice protein

Protein payoff: 16 g per serving

Sunwarrior's claim to fame is using an abundant amount of amino acids. It's also free of GMOs, soy, gluten, dairy, and unnecessary calories. For just one scoop of this flavor-packed drink, you get 80 calories and 16 grams of muscle-molding protein. For a more filling and nutrient-packed meal, double it up! Start your day right with two scoops of this deliciously satisfying chocolate drink for 160 calories and 32 grams of the satiating macronutrient.

$44.99 ($0.95 per serving)

Jarrow Brown Rice

Protein Source: Brown rice protein
Protein payoff: 11 g per serving
Another vegan-friendly option, Jarrow's Brown Rice Protein Concentrate has surprisingly few carbs (3 grams) and 0 grams of sugar per serving, so it's an excellent option for people looking to lose weight. With just 11 grams of protein, however, you might need to supplement it with more protein-rich ingredients: raw almonds, nut butters, or plain low-fat Greek yogurt. The vanilla flavor makes a tasty base for bananas and berries, or blend it with almond butter, cocoa powder, and unsweetened vanilla almond milk for a more decadent-tasting treat.
$9.36 ($0.62 per serving)

Animal-Based Proteins

If you find you're not terribly lactose intolerant, milk proteins are some of the best sources of muscle-building amino acids out there. Milk proteins such as whey and casein have the ability to preserve lean muscle mass and improve metabolic health during weight loss, according to research published in the journal *Nutrition & Metabolism.*

Promix Grass-Fed Whey Protein

Protein source: Grass-fed whey protein concentrate
Protein payoff: 25 g per serving
If you want a fast-acting protein that will stimulate protein synthesis after exercise, go with whey. While a whey protein concentrate has a lower percentage of protein than whey isolate, it contains more bioactive compounds found in the milk fat that positively influence metabolism and immunity. Just make sure it's low-temperature-processed (raw or cold-processed). This method allows the mix to retain many of its fragile immune factors and nutrients, leaving it loaded with the ideal blend of easily absorbed amino acids, anti-inflammatory compounds, essential fats, energy-replenishing carbs,metabolism-boosting peptides, potent antioxidants, and alkaline minerals.

You'll get even more of these nutrients when your powder is made of dairy from pasture-fed cows, which have a higher concentration of inflammation-reducing omega-3 fatty acids and two to five times more conjugated linoleic acid (CLA) than their corn- and grain-fed counterparts. CLA provides a variety of health benefits, like burning fat and maintaining lean body mass. Besides toning your body, these two sources of dietary fat will also improve absorption of key vitamins and carotenoids. Not to mention, grass-fed cows are less likely to be treated with antibiotics than grain-fed cows, meaning you'll have a lower risk of building up antibiotic resistance or gaining unnecessary weight.

$75.99 ($1 per serving)

Naked Casein

Protein source: Micellar casein from U.S. dairy farms
Protein payoff: 26 g per serving
If you're looking to repair and regrow muscle, take some Naked Casein Powder before bed. Casein, as opposed to whey, is digested more slowly (it's the same principle as low-glycemic-index "slow carbs") and stays in the system longer to nourish muscles.

$90.24 ($1.19 per serving)

Mercola Pure Power Protein

Protein source: Grass-fed whey protein concentrate
Protein payoff: 20 g per serving
This product is designed to boost both your fitness level and your overall health. It contains a unique blend of high-quality whey protein, muscle-fueling coconut triglycerides, prebiotic resistant starch, endurance-boosting and blood-sugar-stabilizing chia seeds, and probiotics. Not only can probiotics keep your gut healthy, but also when they're combined with high-quality whey protein, they can enhance muscle development: Probiotics help your body synthesize leucine, a particular branched chain amino acid (BCAA), which you need for muscle building.

$48.97 ($2.18 per serving)

Paleo Protein Pure Egg

Protein source: GMO-free egg whites

Protein payoff: 25.2 g per serving

Whey tends to be the first word when it comes to protein supplementation. But as we've mentioned before, it can cause belly bloat. For a better option that'll help you bulk up only in desirable areas, try egg-white protein, which is naturally low-carb and no-fat. Just like whey, egg-white protein has a complete essential amino acid profile, which promotes optimal recovery from exercise. Want to boost the flavor without artificial additives? Paleo Pure provides a blank slate (it's only egg whites and sunflower lecithin) to add a tablespoon of raw cacao powder to boost your intake of brain-boosting flavonoids while curbing your chocolate cravings.

$44.99 ($1.50 per serving)

Mt. Capra Products Double Bonded Goat Milk Protein

Protein source: Grass-fed goat-milk protein

Protein payoff: 20 g per serving

This powerful protein combines the best of both worlds in protein supplementation through a natural blend of casein and whey proteins. Whey triggers muscle building stimulation while casein inhibits factors that lead to muscle breakdown. Mt. Capra is a small, family-run farm in the Pacific Northwest that uses milk from their own pasture-grazed herd of goats in their powders. If your body doesn't agree with cow milk, goat milk is a great alternative. Even though goat milk still has lactose, the goat-milk proteins are smaller than cow-milk proteins and are thus less prone to disrupting the human digestive system.

$65.23 ($2.17 per serving)

Designer Whey, French Vanilla

Protein Source: Whey full spectrum peptides, whey protein concentrates, whey protein isolate
Protein payoff: 20 g per serving
Like a good pair of designer shoes, Designer Whey lives up to its name. The blend is made up of natural GMO-free whey protein concentrate and GMO-free whey protein isolate. All of the whey from milk is made free of artificial growth hormones and antibiotics. Unlike most animal-based protein powders, this option also provides 3 grams of prebiotic veggie fiber, which helps suppress any hunger between meals.
$44.99 ($0.76 per serving)

How to I.D. a Good Protein Powder

When looking for animal-based protein powders, key on words and phrases like "cold processed," "concentrate," "hormone-free," "grass-fed," "tested low for heavy metals," and "does not contain sucralose or artificial color, flavor, or sweeteners."

Blender Buyer's Guide

A smoothie is just mashed bananas if your blender isn't up to snuff. You need something with enough horsepower to break up ice cubes and turn various fruits and vegetables into drinkable fiber, and you need speed for frothy, belly-filling volume. Your old blender might be just fine. If it's not, its time for an upgrade. Here are a few to consider that we have tried and we like for various reasons. You should be able to find one that's right for you in this list. A good smoothie blender will whip up the 7-Day Smoothie Diet smoothies fast and clean up quickly. (Prices are approximate.)

If you need to mix and run. Invest in a blend-and-go machine if you tend to chug your smoothie while running out the door. Both of these allow you to blend right in your to-go cup. The sets even come with lids to assure you won't have any spills during your commute.

Top Banana: Ninja Nutri Auto-iQ Blender, $120
Budget Buy: Cuisinart Compact-Smoothie Blender, $60

If you're an early riser. Yes, you can blend up a morning smoothie without waking up your household and the one across the street. Sound buffers keep these two quiet even when crushing ice cubes.

Top Banana: Vitamix Quiet One Blender, $1,144
Budget Buy: Jamba Quiet Shield Blender Jar, $149

For the smoothie addict who has everything. Looking for the perfect gift for the ultimate smoothie addict? These unique mix masters are both solid picks. Oster's Mason Jar Blender is perfect for fans of the rustic country trend that's all

the rage right now. The Vitamix is ideal for those who enjoy blending up soups as well as smoothies. In a mere 6 minutes, it can turn cold ingredients into a steaming hot liquid.
Top Banana: Vitamix 5200 Series Blender, $450
Budget Buy: Oster Blend N Go Mason Jar Blender, $30

If you have a retro-style kitchen. Farm chic and retro-inspired kitchens are endearing and enduring, and these fashion-forward blenders are the perfect accessories to complete the vintage look.
Top Banana: Smeg Retro Style Blender, $250
Budget Buy: Nostalgia Retro Series Blender, $46

For the tiny kitchen. Is your kitchen only slightly roomier than the galley of a commuter jet? Then take a look at these tiny powerhouses: The Bella Blender comes with grinding and blending blades and various-size blending cups and to-go lids. The five-inch-wide NutriBullet is just as versatile and comes complete with various types of blades, cups, lip rings, and lids. It even shreds, chops, and grinds.
Top Banana: Magic Bullet NutriBullet 12-Piece High-Speed Blender/Mixer System, $86
Budget Buy: Bella 12-Piece Rocket Blender, $24

If you never have time to clean. If you love smoothies, but hate cleaning gritty protein out of from under the blades, these blenders will make your day: They auto-clean. The Vitamix handles crud in just 60 seconds. Just add soap. Both have preset buttons for creations like smoothies, hot soups, frozen desserts, and purees.
Top Banana: Vitamix Professional Series 750, $599
Budget Buy: Breville Boss Easy to Use Superblender, $395

CHAPTER

4

7 Days of Hunger-Busting Smoothie Recipes

KNOWING EXACTLY WHAT you are going to eat for your meals and snacks is one of the most powerful ways to lose weight and stay healthy. It's when we don't have a plan in place that we often get into trouble. You're hungry for breakfast but don't know what to have, and time is ticking by before you rush out the door, so you grab a bowl of sugary cereal or, worse, a chocolate-dipped doughnut from the box on the kitchen counter. At lunchtime or snack time, you didn't bring anything from home, so you hit a fast-food restaurant or a vending machine.

The Smoothie Rule—one in the morning and one in the afternoon—means you have two fewer decisions to make today. Hooray! You know what you're going to have. You just need to pick the flavor. And this chapter will give you those options—heavier smoothies designed for breakfast, and lighter afternoon smoothies made for giving you a burst of late-day energy. At the end of this chapter, you'll find other smoothie recipes with specific health benefits that you can use after you complete the 7-Day Smoothie Diet challenge.

The breakfast smoothies recommended here are typically made with healthy fats and proteins to keep your belly satisfied until lunchtime. These carry anywhere from 250 to 500 calories. You'll also find some smoothie bowl recipes in the mix in case you'd prefer to eat something with a spoon instead of a straw a day or two during the 7-Day Smoothie Diet. Fats used in the recipes include nut butters, seeds, avocado, extra-virgin olive oil, and coconut oil. The first four on that list are those heart-healthy monounsaturated fats that you've heard so much about in the past 15 years. Coconut oil is a saturated fat, a specific kind called a medium chain triglyceride that some studies show can aid in weight loss. Like the mono fats, coconut oil is satiating, too. And it has a pleasant scent and taste. However, coconut oil does raise LDL (bad) cholesterol, which is why the American Heart Association does not advocate eating coconut oil. Coconut oil also raises HDL, the good cholesterol, so it's not at all a doom-and-gloom ingredient. As long as you don't cook with coconut oil all the time and drink coconut oil smoothies every day, we think you won't see your LDL levels go up on this plan. But if you do currently have high LDL cholesterol, stick to the smoothies made with the monounsaturated fats.

Breakfast Smoothies

Note: Blend all ingredients together unless indicated.

---

1. Almond Crush

Savory almond butter is a protein powerhouse that clobbers hunger and builds fat-burning lean muscle. The tear-shaped nuts from which it's made actually contain a compound that reduces the amount of fat absorbed by the body. In fact, a study published in the *Journal of the American Heart Association* showed that eating just 1.5 ounces of almonds daily led to a reduction in belly and leg fat.

1 Tbsp. almond butter
½ orange, peeled
½ frozen banana
1 cup spinach, tightly packed
½ cup unsweetened almond milk
1 tsp. flaxseed oil
1 scoop vanilla plant-based protein powder
3 ice cubes
Water to blend (if needed)

Makes 1 serving.

Per serving: 330 calories, 9 g fat, 29 g carbohydrates, 6 g fiber, 31 g protein

---

2. PB & JP

1 cup mixed frozen blueberries and blackberries
2 Tbsp. no-sugar-added peanut butter
¼ cup vanilla protein powder
2 Tbsp. rolled oats
1 cup unsweetened almond milk

Makes 1 serving.

Per serving: 417 calories, 11 g fat, 41 g carbohydrates, 6 g fiber, 41 g protein

3. Yo-oatmeal

The oats plump in your stomach, keeping your hunger away for hours.

½ cup blueberries
½ cup unsweetened oatmeal, cooked
½ cup Greek yogurt
1 tsp. chia seeds
Water as needed to thin consistency

Makes 1 serving.

Per serving: 271 calories, 4 g fat, 44 g carbohydrates, 7 g fiber, 18 g protein

4. Mega Greens Smoothie

Avocado adds creaminess to any smoothie, plus a healthy dose of monounsaturated fat, which helps stabilize blood sugar and burn fat.

½ cup plain nonfat Greek yogurt
1 cup spinach
1 medium frozen banana, cut up
½ cup frozen pineapple chunks
¼ avocado
1 Tbsp. parsley
2 tsp. extra-virgin olive oil
Water as needed to thin consistency.

Makes 1 serving.

Per serving: 347 calories, 15 g fat, 45 g carbohydrates, 7 g fiber, 15 g protein

5. Chocolate Peanut Butter Power House

Tofu is ideal for adding a silky texture and some satiating protein—plus serious fat burning. Tofu is packed with isoflavones, a type of antioxidant, and it's also particularly high

in fat-blasting genistein, a compound that acts directly on obesity genes, helping to turn them off and reduce the storage of body fat.

1 banana, sliced
⅓ cup tofu, cut into cubes
½ cup spinach
1 cup unsweetened almond milk
¼ cup plain Greek yogurt
1 Tbsp. creamy peanut butter
2 tsp. local honey
2 tsp. cocoa powder
1 tsp. chia seeds
5 ice cubes

- Add banana slices, tofu cubes, and spinach to a blender. Top with ½ cup of almond milk and Greek yogurt. Blend on high until smooth. Add peanut butter, honey, cocoa powder, chia seeds, and the rest of the milk and blend until smooth.

Makes 2 servings.

Per serving: 301 calories, 9 g fat, 45 g carbohydrates, 5 g fiber, 19 g protein

---

6. Walnut Mint Chip

Walnuts are a perfect weight-loss food. Their fiber and fat combine to make you feel fuller longer. One review of 31 clinical trials found that study participants whose diets included walnuts lost about 1.4 extra pounds and half an inch from their waists. The peppermint oil, banana, and cacao in this smoothie overpowers any of the bitterness you might detect from walnuts.

¼ cup walnuts
½ cup unsweetened almond milk
1 medium banana, greenish skin, not quite ripe
¾ cup baby spinach
¼ cup fresh mint leaves

½ tsp. peppermint oil
4 ice cubes
1 Tbsp. cacao nibs to garnish
½ cup water (if it's too thick for you)

- Save a few mint leaves and some cacao nibs for a garnish, then put the rest of the ingredients in a powerful blender and blend until smooth. Add water if too thick.

Makes 1 serving.

Per serving: 350 calories, 27 g fat, 22 g carbohydrates, 7 g fiber, 7 g protein

---

7. Kiwi, Kefir, and Kale

Think of kefir as a drinkable yogurt. It delivers high amounts of calcium, magnesium, folate, vitamins B2 and B12, plus gut-friendly enzymes and probiotics. And it's often well tolerated by people who have problems with lactose.

1 cup kale, chopped, packed
1 cup full-fat kefir
1 medium frozen banana
1 Tbsp. almond butter
1 kiwi, peeled

Makes 1 serving.

Per serving: 425 calories, 18 g fat, 58 g carbohydrates, 8 g fiber, 18 g protein

---

8. Bunny and Banana

2 carrots, peeled
½ frozen banana
1 cup unsweetened almond milk
1 tsp. fresh ginger, grated
1 scoop vanilla plant-based protein powder
1 tsp. ground flaxseed

Makes 1 serving.

Per serving: 280 calories, 5 g fat, 33 g carbohydrate, 8 g fiber, 24 g protein

9. Matcha Berry Overnight Oats Bowl

1 medium banana
½ cup uncooked oats
½ cup coconut milk
¼ cup unsweetened almond milk
1 Tbsp. chia seeds
1 tsp. powdered matcha green tea
Pinch of sea salt
3 fresh strawberries, sliced
⅓ cup fresh blueberries

- Mash the banana with a fork, then combine with oats, coconut milk, almond milk, chia seeds, matcha powder, and salt in a plastic or glass container with a lid. Cover and refrigerate overnight. In the morning, stir the contents into a cereal bowl and top with the strawberries and blueberries.

Makes 1 serving.

Per serving: 440 calories, 20 g fat, 68 g carbohydrates, 10 g fiber, 9 g protein

10. The Blueberry Granola Bowl

1 cup frozen blueberries
½ cup unsweetened almond milk
1½ scoops whey- or plant-based protein powder
2 Tbsp. almond butter
1 tsp. vanilla extract

For the Topping

½ cup fresh blueberries or strawberries
¼ cup vanilla granola
2 Tbsp. sliced almonds
2 tsp. hemp seeds
1 tsp. cinnamon

Makes 2 servings.

Per serving: 372 calories, 17 g fat, 32 g carbohydrates, 7 g fiber, 25 g protein

Afternoon Smoothies

1. The Coffee Break Smoothie

This one will clear the afternoon cobwebs and get you through the rest of the day. It's also a solid smoothie to drink after or even before exercise. Fiber-packed flaxseed contains more inflammation-fighting omega-3 fatty acids than other fat sources. That means it's good for reducing inflammation and helping with post-exercise muscle recovery. Flaxseed is highly sensitive and easily oxidized, so for the greatest health benefit, buy whole flaxseed and grind it just before adding to your smoothie.

½ cup brewed coffee
(use decaf if caffeine late in the day affects your sleep)
½ large banana, cut into chunks
½ cup plain Greek yogurt
½ Tbsp. ground flaxseed
1 tsp. local honey
¼ tsp. cinnamon
¼ tsp. grated nutmeg (optional)

Makes 1 serving.

Per serving: 135 calories, 1.3 g fat, 21 g carbohydrates, 2.4 g fiber, 9 g protein

2. Orange Aid

This sweet smoothie is like a multivitamin in a glass. Loaded with vitamin C from the orange and lemon, it also contains immune-system-boosting ginger, plus folate and vitamin K from the spinach.

1 orange, peeled
1 banana, peeled
½ -in. chunk of ginger

1 handful baby spinach
Juice of 1 lemon
1 Tbsp. hempseed
1 cup water
4 ice cubes

Makes 2 servings.

Per serving: 112 calories, 2 g fat, 22 g carbohydrates, 3 g fiber, 2 g protein

---

3. Awesome Tea Party

Brewable green tea is good. Matcha is much better because it's a fine powder made from young, green tea leaves that delivers a much higher concentration of antioxidant catechins, including EGCG, a metabolism booster that breaks down belly fat cells. You can add matcha green tea powder to many smoothie recipes to reap the health benefits. This recipe uses banana, vanilla-flavored protein powder, and cinnamon to mask the distinct flavor of matcha, which some don't care for.

½ cup baby spinach, loosely packed
½ frozen banana
1 tsp. matcha green tea powder
1 tsp. ground cinnamon
1 scoop vanilla plant-based protein powder
Water to blend (optional)

Makes 1 serving.

Per serving: 226 calories, 1 g fat, 25 g carbohydrates, 6 g fiber, 26 g protein

---

4. The Cinnamon Solution

Studies haven proven cinnamon's power as a blood sugar stabilizer. Adding a teaspoon of the spice to a carb-rich meal prevents insulin spikes that drive overeating, according to research in the *American Journal of Clinical Nutrition*. That makes this smoothie one heck of a belly-fat buster. Bonus: This

smoothie is an easy way to add collards to your diet. These dark greens are among the world's healthiest foods, a great source of carotenoids, manganese, vitamin C, vitamin E, copper, folate, niacin, and even omega-3s.

1 generous handful of collard greens
1 pear, chopped
1 medium apple, chopped
1 tsp. cinnamon
1 Tbsp. plant-based protein powder
1 cup water
1 cup ice

Makes 2 servings.

Per serving: 150 calories, 1 g fat, 32 g carbohydrates, 12 g fiber, 6 g protein

---

5. Almonds and Strawberries

5 medium strawberries
1 cup unsweetened almond milk
½ cup low-fat plain Greek yogurt
5 ice cubes

Makes 1 serving.

Per serving: 167 calories, 6 g fat, 11 g carbohydrates, 2 g fiber, 16 g protein

---

6. Carrot with a Kick

Ginger, the spicy root known for its ability to quell nausea and other bellyaches, combines with fresh carrots and lemon for a refreshing pick-me-up.

2 oz. carrots
½ apple, chopped
½ cucumber chopped
Juice of half a lemon
½ -in. ginger
1 Tbsp. hemp seeds

1 cup water
1 cup ice

Makes 1 serving.

Per serving: 103 calories, 1.6 g fat, 19 g carbohydrates, 4 g fiber, 3 g protein

---

7. Fruit Loopers

½ frozen banana
1 medium apple, cored and chopped
1 scoop whey protein powder
½ avocado
½ cup strawberries, sliced
1 tsp. chia seeds
½ tsp. grated fresh ginger
½ cup coconut milk

Makes 2 servings.

Per serving: 300 calories, 15 g fat, 26 g carbohydrates, 12 g fiber, 10 g protein

---

8. The Cabbage Patch

This smoothie packs a garden full of superfoods into a glass, including purple cabbage, a cruciferous vegetable that, like broccoli and cauliflower, has strong cancer-preventive properties. It's also rich in vitamin C, fiber, and omega-3s for brain and heart health.

¾ cup purple cabbage, roughly chopped
½ cup frozen blueberries
1 small Crispin or Granny Smith apple, cored and cubed
1 Tbsp. chia seeds
½ cup coconut water

Makes 1 serving.

Per serving: 245 calories, 5 g fat, 45 g carbohydrates, 12 g fiber, 6 g protein

9. Cinnamon Swirl

A creamy, satisfying, dairy-free shake that'll clobber midafternoon hunger pangs. Add a few ice cubes to make it frothier.

½ banana
1 tsp. cinnamon
1 Tbsp. ground chia seeds
1 cup vanilla almond milk
1 scoop plain or vanilla plant-based protein powder

Makes 1 serving.

Per serving: 262 calories, 4 g fat, 32 g carbohydrates, 5 g fiber, 25 g protein

10. Cucumber, Collards, and Cranberries

1½ oz. collard greens
1 medium apple, peel on, chopped
2 oz. cranberries
1 small cucumber, chopped
1 Tbsp. flaxseeds
1 Tbsp. beet powder or dried hibiscus (optional)
1 cup water
1 cup ice

Makes 2 servings.

Per serving: 95 calories, 1.5 g fat, 20 g carbohydrates, 7 g fiber, 1 g protein

For more smoothie recipes, see page 131.

HACK YOUR SMOOTHIES

Keep some of these add-ins on hand to concoct smoothies that will crank up your metabolism and help you burn more fat.

- **Almond butter**
- **Almond milk and other nut milks**
- **Avocado**
- **Apples**
- **Beets**
- **Black, green, and white tea**
- **Cayenne pepper**
- **Cinnamon**
- **Coconut milk**
- **Coconut oil**
- **Coconut water**
- **Collard greens**
- **Cottage cheese**
- **Cow's milk**
- **Cucumber**
- **Flaxseeds and flaxseed oil**
- **Frozen fruit, mixed**
- **Frozen bananas**
- **Ginger**
- **Grapes**
- **Greek yogurt**
- **Kale**
- **Kefir**
- **Kiwifruit**
- **Lemons and Limes**
- **Matcha powder**

HACK YOUR SMOOTHIES (Continued)

- Mango
- Olive oil
- Oranges
- Papaya
- Parsley
- Pears
- Protein powder
- Raw local honey
- Raspberries
- Spinach
- Strawberries
- Swiss chard
- Tiger nuts (trendy tubers high in resistant starch)

CHAPTER

5

Rule #2
Eat Extra-Filling Foods

THIS IS AN important weight-loss principle because it works hand-in-hand with Rule #1: Drink smoothies. Choosing the right foods—healthy, extra-filling foods—to eat for breakfast, lunch, and dinner is the best way to lose weight and energize your body most efficiently. Consider this auto analogy:

Let's say you weren't a woman or man, but an expensive automobile, like a Porsche or a BMW. Pick the ride you want to be. Now, a car like you usually packs a high-performance engine under the hood. Not to get too technical, but what makes these engines special is their high compression ratio, meaning the air and fuel mixture in the cylinders becomes extra compressed for more power.

You can use regular unleaded gas in these engines, but that'll typically cause pre-ignition of the fast-burning fuel and trigger knocking and diminished performance and fuel efficiency. Ever hear your car knock? That's what's happening. That's why manufacturers of performance cars recommend you use premium fuel, with an octane rating of 91 or 93 versus regular gas's 87. What's so special about the more expensive high-octane fuel? It doesn't burn prematurely under high piston pressure. You get more power, no knocks, better efficiency.

Let's turn the ignition off and go back to being you. Your body is similar to that hot set of wheels in that it runs better on better fuel. Better fuel is food that burns more slowly and steadily, keeping your blood sugar stable, no knocks, er, spikes that quickly dip and drive cravings and overeating. Better food is high in protein, fiber-rich carbohydrates, and a little fat. All three types of macronutrients are digested more slowly than fast-burning carbohydrates like simple sugars. They stick with you longer, they even out the flow of glucose into your bloodstream that powers your action, and they won't make you fat.

Cookies Crumbled

To understand how proteins and fiber-rich carbs affect your body differently from sugary carbs, grab a cookie. Eat the cookie. Delicious, isn't it? Want another? Of course you do. (But push away that bag before it's too late!)

Now, if you had a nice piece of grilled chicken breast, a few raw broccoli florets, or a chunk of cheese, you probably wouldn't react with the same ravenous reach for more.

Why is that so? Why can't you eat just one cookie but it's easy enough to take a pass on more broccoli? It's because there's nothing worthwhile inside that cookie that tells your body, "That's enough. I'm full." Cookies are nothing more than little pancakes of sugar and salt, as addictive as a controlled substance. There's little protein or fiber to stall the injection of glucose into your bloodstream. When your blood sugar dips, you become hungry again. And the cycle continues.

The 7-Day Smoothie Diet strategy keeps that fat-forming scenario from happening.

Save 100 Calories (or More) Per Meal

Easy tweaks that can help you shed more pounds.

Baby steps can take you a long way. Think about it: A seemingly insignificant move, like not adding croutons to your salad, can slash 100 calories from your meal. That can add up to a pound of weight loss over the course of a month of eating without going hungry, without doing extra exercise, and while still eating the foods you love.

Here are some other painless ways to slash (at least) 100 calories:

- **Eat tuna that's been packed in water instead of oil.**
- **Swap out cheese on your hamburger for lettuce, tomato, and onion.**
- **Use one fewer tablespoon of butter on your baked potato or bread.**
- **Remove the skin from chicken.**
- **Eat an open-faced turkey sandwich on one slice of whole-wheat bread instead of using two slices of bread.**
- **Replace the mayonnaise on that sandwich with zero-calorie yellow mustard.**

- Go with chives, not cheese, on your scrambled eggs.
- Sip seltzer with lemon slices, not soda.
- Use olive oil spray (5 calories) instead of a tablespoon of olive oil (120 calories).
- Instead of spaghetti, use zoodles (spiralized veggies).
- Order Canadian bacon in place of sausage or bacon with your scrambled egg breakfast.
- Bake a homemade pizza with half the cheese.
- Pour a serving of pretzels into a bowl instead of eating from the bag.

"What Should I Eat?"

How many times a day do you subconsciously ask yourself that question? How many times a week? When you don't have a good, quick answer, that can spell trouble for your waistline. Because when you don't know what to eat when hungry, it's very hard to eat mindfully. Hunger hormones hijack your brain and send you hunting for something to satisfy your cravings fast: you zero in on fast food, easy-to-grab salty snacks, or a quick calorie-dense meal.

The 7-Day Smoothie Diet provides the answers to the question, "What should I eat?" so you're not searching for the solution. Rules 1 and 2 ensure that you get the right mix of nutrients you need for all-day energy: Two delicious smoothies, one in the morning, one in the afternoon, and a lunch and a dinner made up of extra-filling foods guarantees that you get something good in your belly every few hours. You never feel as if you are "starving." Rules 1 and 2 eliminate the guesswork at the heart of our poor eating habits.

But, you may be thinking, what are "extra-filling foods"? Is it a quarter-pound cheeseburger with French fries? That sounds filling, right? Yes, but it isn't. Extra-filling foods satisfy your hunger for a long time. That burger and those fries, though high in calories, do not stick with you. Here's why: For one, that burger meat probably has some trans fat in it. Trans fats cause inflammation in the gut, which can disrupt appetite-regulating chemicals that signal you to stop eating. The bun and the condiments contain high fructose corn syrup, the manmade sugars responsible for insulin spikes that then drop, decreasing energy and triggering stronger hunger pangs. And all that salt. The high level of sodium in burgers and fries and other fast foods causes dehydration, which we often mistake for, you guessed it, hunger.

So, you see, calorie-dense foods—pizza, spaghetti and meatballs, grilled cheese sandwiches, chocolate frosted cake, cookies and more—are not extra-filling. Instead, they are extra fattening.

No, an "extra-filling food" is very different. It's one that combines high protein with healthy fats, fiber, and water. The last two ingredients—fiber and water—tend to make the food low in energy density. That's the kind of food that will fill you up and stick with you. And help you lose weight.

Many years ago, Australian researchers conducted a study in which they gave participants different types of foods to eat and then asked them to rate their satiety levels over the two hours after taking the last bite. Each portion contained exactly the same number of calories, 240, so the scientists could determine which of the foods tested would work best for keeping people feeling fuller for longer. Have a look at the top foods on the researchers "satiety index" list. All are rich in at least one if not more of the essential components in our definition of an "extra-filling food."

Apples—High in water and fiber, low in energy density.
Beans—Beans and legumes contain protein and lots of fiber, both of which are processed more slowly in the stomach, extending feelings of fullness.
Beef—Lean sirloin steak versus ground chuck is rich in satiating protein. One study in the *International Journal of Obesity* found that people who had a high-protein lunch ate 12 percent less at dinner when compared with a high-carbohydrate lunch.
Fish—Not the breaded and deep-fried stuff. We're talking about a nice thick fillet of tuna, salmon, halibut, bass, cod, or trout, baked, broiled, or grilled. Fish is the most satiating of the proteins on the satiety index, and it comes with heart-healthy fats, too.
Eggs—One of best low-calorie sources of protein you can eat, eggs make a terrific protein around which to build a healthy, extra-filling lunch or dinner.
Oatmeal—Of course it's a good source of fiber (4 grams in just one cup), but did you know that it provides more protein per serving any another other grain? Mix in some seeds and nuts to add an extra dose of fiber and satiating fat.
Popcorn—This snack food ranked much higher on the satiety list than pretzels or potato chips because it's a lot of air and fiber. It's bulky, so it makes you chew, which spurs satiety, and its fiber expands in your belly. Because it's so high in volume, yet so low in energy, calorie for calorie, it's one of the most filling foods you can eat. Just opt for the air-popped version and stay away from microwaved popcorn, which tends to be high in oil, which elevates the calorie content significantly.
Salad—If it's not your main course, feel free to add a salad to any lunch or dinner recipe suggestion in this book. Why?

Salads are bulky, full of water and fiber, and low in calories, so they fill you up for less. But avoid drowing them in high-calorie dressings.

Soup—Researchers at Penn State University found that people who consumed soup twice a day lost more weight and kept off an average of 16 pounds over the course of a year compared with people who didn't eat soup. Broth-based soups that are chunky with vegetables, beans, or chicken will fill you up best.

Get Moving After Eating

Muscles that are moving soak up glucose from your bloodstream more quickly and effectively than muscles that are sedentary. So anytime you have something to eat, have some exercise for dessert. It doesn't have to be much. Just getting up from the table and talking a walk can help. Hit the stairs. Put away the laundry. Do a few body weight exercises. Anything physical will give the blood sugar a place to go.

Focus on Fullness

It sounds a little counterintuitive—eating more can help you weigh less. But the extra-filling foods strategy works so well because it takes care of the problem that undermines so many other diet strategies: sacrifice. Limiting your diet, as most diets require, usually backfires because you end up hungry, even hangry (hungry + angry) and you toss up your hands and go back to eating Pizza Hut's cheese-filled crust pizzas.

Penn State nutritionist Barbara Rolls, PhD, is a pioneer in focusing on fullness to lose weight and keep it off. Rolls believes one of the key paths to losing weight is filling up on foods that aren't heavy with calories. These foods are what she calls high-volume foods, high in air, water, and fiber, that make your belly expand. Her research led to a weight loss approach she calls Volumetrics, about which she has written several popular diet books. The concept is simple: For the calories you would consume in just two bites of a bacon cheeseburger, you could enjoy, say, a big bowl of minestrone soup. Which one would satisfy your more, two bites of burger or a whole bowl of soup? Second question: Would you be able to stop at just two bites of cheeseburger?

So, you see, by mindfully choosing a high-volume, extra-filling food over a calorie-dense one, you've created a win-win: You eat more food and lose weight. This is why focusing on fullness is such an important part of the 7-Day Smoothie Diet. By planning your meals so that they virtually guarantee fullness and satisfaction, you do not have to make sacrifices or fear the gnawing hunger pangs that send you in search of your kids' leftover Halloween candy stash.

What's high volume, high-water-content food? Take a look at the last two entries on the Australian researchers' satiety list: salads and soups. What do they have in common? Lots of vegetables, lots of water, lots of fiber.

How many soups and salads do you see on your prep day food logs? If the kind of diet you recorded is full of energy-dense processed foods, switching to high-water-volume foods like vegetable salads and soups will virtually guarantee rapid weight loss. You don't have to think much about what you're eating. Just cook up the lunch and dinner recipes listed in Chapter 9. They were selected to deliver low-calorie, high-fiber vegetables and grains, and satiating lean proteins and healthy fats. And if you'd like to supplement those meals with even more fresh vegetables to fill your belly, by all means—go right ahead. Start chopping up these watery wonders, listed according to their percentage of water content by weight:

- **Cucumber: 97%**
- **Raw radishes: 95%**
- **Celery: 95%**
- **Watermelon: 91%**
- **Raw broccoli: 89%**
- **Peaches: 89%**
- **Yogurt: 88%**
- **Raw carrots: 88%**
- **Plums: 87%**
- **Apples: 86%**

There's something you should notice about the vegetables and fruits above and those on the satiety list. They are whole, single-ingredient foods. If you ever wonder if a food qualifies as "extra-filling," ask yourself, "Is it mostly made up of whole foods or is it processed?" The answer will be apparent. And you'll have your solution to the conundrum: What should I eat?

For years nutritionists and weight-loss coaches have advised their clients never to go food shopping on an empty stomach. Have something: a bowl of oatmeal, a smoothie and scrambled eggs, a banana slathered with peanut butter. Why? Because when you're hungry, you'll face much greater temptation to fill your shopping cart with candy, chips, cookies, and other baked goods. Why do you think the checkout aisle is always bordered by racks filled with Snickers and Hershey's bars, boxes of Slim Jims, and little bags of trail mix? Those calorie-dense snacks are there to tempt you when you're most vulnerable—hungry and faced with the realization that you have to drive home and put away all those groceries before you can eat.

When you're feeling full, you're not obsessed with filling the void in your belly. You're able to think and plan and make much smarter food choices. Have a meal and then go food shopping, and you'll be much more likely to fill your cart with healthy, low-calorie whole foods.

Do you see the pattern here? By keeping your body fueled with smoothies (high-protein, high-water-volume nutrition) and extra-filling foods (high-protein, high-fiber, high-water-volume, low-energy nutrition), you will automatically reduce the number of calories you consume during those meals, and you'll delete calorie-dense processed foods that are causing weight gain in the first place.

Best of all, you'll be establishing a habit of eating only those highly nutritious foods that support a lean, healthy, fit body.

Eat Your Drinks

Easy ways to get more extra-filling, high-water content, low-calorie foods.

- Combine a mix of fresh or frozen chopped fruit for a fruit salad.
- Add a twist to your fruit salad with lime juice, balsamic vinegar, or some fresh herbs like mint or basil.
- Make fruit kebabs with fresh-cut mixed fruit.
- Put just about any veggie—or fruits like peaches or pineapple—on the grill.
- Make a tropical green smoothie with mango, pineapple, banana, and spinach.
- Use sliced cucumber, carrots, or bell peppers with dips or salsas instead of chips.
- Make a refreshing summer salad topped with fresh berries or peaches.
- Substitute for rice with grated or finely chopped cauliflower.
- Puree frozen bananas to make a very simple "ice cream."

CHAPTER

6

Rule #3

Smack Down Hunger with Cravings Crushers

CRAVINGS ARE POWERFUL FORCES. A bowl of M&Ms or Hershey's Kisses pulls us toward it like a high-powered magnet. You too? We've all been there. It's like we are weaklings with no strength or willpower to fight this invisible tug of instant gratification. We yield, and feel terrible about it even while licking the last smudge of milk chocolate off our cheeks.

Yes, cravings are powerful. But they are not insurmountable. In fact, they are pretty easy to head off, to crush even. You're stronger than a food craving. Much. You just need to recognize the power within you to break its grip. It also helps to use some tricks, call 'em cheats if you wish, to outsmart your brain's fixation on those chocolates, doughnuts, scoops of ice cream, slices of cake—you fill in the blank.

In a way, a craving is like a sour mood. If you're in a funk, a really bad mood, it's very difficult to knock yourself out of wallowing in your anger and misery. But a bad mood doesn't have to be perpetual. You can get out of it by breaking the spell.

Several years ago researchers discovered that you can improve your mood simply by forcing a smile. The study called "Grin and Bear It: The Influence of Manipulated Positive Facial Expression on the Stress Response," was published in the prestigious journal *Psychological Science*. In the study, researchers actually used chopsticks to manipulate the mouths of 169 participants into either a neutral expression, a pleasant standard smile, or an ear-to-ear grin. It turned out that forcing the lips into a broad grin caused the participants' moods to improve.

The point is, you have more power than you think to manipulate and change your long-standing habits, intense cravings, and even your mood, which plays a huge role in eating behaviors. Try these tools and techniques to empower your resolve.

CRAVINGS CRUSHER:
Eat Yogurt.

Feeling down can jumpstart emotional eating. Head it off by having a small cup of Greek yogurt. The protein in the yogurt will elevate levels of mood-boosting neurotransmitters while feeding your gut probiotics, which research has linked to improved mood.

CRAVINGS CRUSHER:
Run for 30 Minutes.

Scientists at Loughborough University in England say running for that length of time curbs hunger by increasing production of the appetite-suppressing peptide YY and decreasing the appetite stimulant ghrelin.

CRAVINGS CRUSHER:
Jump Rope.

The bouncing motion disturbs the digestive track, which can quell the impulse to eat, say British researchers.

CRAVINGS CRUSHER:
Drink Cold Water.

Did you know that 60 percent of the time we inappropriately respond to thirst by eating instead of drinking? So says a study in the journal *Physiology & Behavior*. Experts believe the mistake stems from the fact that the same part of our brain controls hunger and thirst, and sometimes it mixes up the signals. Not only will keeping a water bottle around help you respond to thirst correctly, but chugging water can help you feel full and keep your metabolism humming. In fact, if you drink ice-cold water, your body will burn a few extra calories heating that water up once it's inside you!

CRAVINGS CRUSHER:
Close the Kitchen at Night.

Limiting when you eat is, in some ways, just as important as limiting what you eat. According to a recent study published in *Cell Metabolism*, mice that engaged in "time-restricted feeding" (TRF)—eating only during a nine- to

12-hour period of activity and abstaining from food for the 12-hour sedentary, overnight period—showed signs of reversing the progression of metabolic disease and type 2 diabetes. In fact, the experiment showed that eating under a time-restricted feeding schedule effectively stymied weight gain even when used with high-calorie, high-fructose, and high-fat diets, and was still effective even when the TRF was disrupted on the weekends (which is great to know, because how many times have you given in to a late-night craving on a Saturday?). In other words, stay away from the pantry from 8 p.m. to 8 a.m.

CRAVINGS CRUSHER:
Chickpea "Chips."

If you have an insatiable craving for a salty snack, have one, but make it this one: spicy chickpea "chips."

2 15-oz. cans chickpeas, drained
1 Tbsp. extra-virgin olive oil
2 tsp. Cajun spice mix
1 tsp. granulated garlic
½ tsp. dried oregano, crumbled

- Preheat oven to 450°F.
- Place the chickpeas and olive oil in a resealable plastic bag. Close the bag and shake until the chickpeas are well coated with oil.
- Place the oiled chickpeas on a rimmed cookie sheet and then roast, occasionally turning with a spatula until golden and crisp, about 45 minutes. Transfer the roasted chickpeas to a serving bowl and toss with the remaining ingredients.

Makes 4 servings.

Per serving: 235 calories, 3 g fat (2 g saturated), 71 mg sodium, 4 g fiber, 5 g protein

CRAVINGS CRUSHER:
Stay Busy.

Downtime can be bad for your waistline. One study concluded that most people eat when they are bored to escape monotony rather than to increase satisfaction. Keep busy with a hobby like learning to play guitar or piano, knitting, or doing a craft project. Pop packing bubbles if it will keep your hands out of the chip bag. Research shows that cravings usually last between three and 10 minutes, so doing something to distract yourself for 10 minutes or so may be all you need to crush a craving. Put down the candy bar and take a walk instead. You'll feel great when you get back.

CRAVINGS CRUSHER:
Call a Friend.

Take a few minutes to connect with someone you care about. Your spirits will be lifted, and your mind will be distracted from thoughts of eating. Chances are your call will perk them up, too.

CRAVINGS CRUSHER:
Gnaw on Some Celery.

High-water-content, low-calorie foods that are crunchy, like celery, carrots, broccoli, and cauliflower help boost your energy and reduce cravings for sugar and processed foods.

CRAVINGS CRUSHER:
Swig a Shot of Kefir.

Eat This, Not That! readers have told us that fermented drinks like kefir reduce or eliminate cravings for sugar and baked goods. Give it a shot. The next time you have a craving, take a two-ounce shot of your favorite probiotic liquid, like kefir or CocoBiotic. You'll be amazed at how the sour taste of the fermented drink relieves the desire for sugar and processed foods.

CRAVINGS CRUSHER:
Meditate.

Meditation can help chase away cravings by helping to reduce stress and focus your mind. In 2015, Sara Lazar, a neuroscientist at Harvard Medical School and Massachusetts General Hospital, discovered that meditation not only has the power to reduce stress, but it can change the brain by increasing gray matter in the auditory and sensory cortex. Stress creates the hormone cortisol, which increases your blood sugar. This is a vicious cycle that damages your adrenals and creates sugar cravings. Adding a short meditation before meals can help you relax, which means better digestion and absorption of nutrients.

CRAVINGS CRUSHER:
Indulge in a Spoonful.

According to one Stanford University study, we all have a unique "taste-health balance point" that allows us to feel satisfied with a certain ratio of indulgent food to healthy food. Specifically, the study concluded that most people only need about a quarter of their "vice–virtue bundle" to be made up of the vice (let's say it's ice cream), and three quarters can be the good stuff (apple and peanut butter); this ratio was shown to encourage people to feel satisfied and eat more of the healthy stuff. So go ahead and let yourself have some French fries with dinner, but be sure to also have a couple extra bites of salad for the perfect balance.

CHAPTER

7

Rule #4
Get Moving!

IF SOMEONE SHOT a video of you during your 15 or so waking hours, what would it look like, an action movie or a film about a particular South American mammal noted for slowness of movement? If you're like most Americans, your film would fall somewhere in between, but a lot closer to a documentary of the three-toed sloth than, say, the latest Avengers movie.

Recent surveys estimate that 80 percent of American adults do not meet the government's call for 150 minutes of aerobic and muscle strengthening activity per week. The Physical Activity Council reports that the number of totally sedentary adults continues to rise; about 83 million Americans age six and over, roughly 28 percent of the population, did not participate in any of 104 specific physical activities in the last calendar year.

We all need to increase the movement in our days. We spend far too much time sitting (7.7 hours, on average) often staring at a TV or a computer screen (2 hours a day on average). You already know this, and you have a good idea where you stand, er, sit. Even if you aren't a fan of formal exercise, you know you should be moving more each day.

One reason that we are incorporating a plan to get moving into the 7-Day Smoothie Diet challenge is that studies show that combining healthier eating habits (reducing sugars and calories) with more exercise appears to be the best way for people to improve their lifestyles. Feeling fitter can make you happier and less stressed, reducing the urge to eat for emotional reasons. We know that when we're eating healthfully, we tend to have more motivation to exercise.

The physical and mental health benefits of aerobic fitness are broad and deep. You've heard these before, but let's tick off a few to jog our memories:

Exercise strengthens your heart. Boosting your heart rate regularly can reduce your risk of cardiovascular disease and stroke. Increasing your heart rate through exercise helps to make your blood vessels more pliable, less stiff, lowering high blood pressure.

Exercise eases depression. Some studies comparing people with depression taking antidepressant medication to depressed people who followed an aerobic exercise program showed that exercise alone was just as effective as pills at improving depression symptoms. But please consult your doctor before considering abandoning your medication. It is important to stop taking antidepressants only under a physician's guidance.

Exercise boosts mood. Even if you aren't suffering depression, physical activity can lift your spirits. Exercise triggers the release of feel-good brain chemicals called endorphins. Give it a self-test. Go for a brisk walk this afternoon and see how you feel. We'll bet you'll feel less stressed after your walk, especially if you did it outside. A study in *Environmental Science & Technology* recently found that you're also more likely to report a greater sense of pleasure, enthusiasm, and self-esteem and lower sense of depression, tension, and fatigue simply by walking in nature compared to walking on a dreary treadmill.

Exercise may extend your life. Consider this: According to the Centers for Disease Control and Prevention, exercising for one hour a day makes you 40 percent less likely to die early than someone who only exercises for 30 minutes once a week.

Altering your walking pace and direction can cause your body to burn up to 20 percent more calories than just maintaining a steady speed.

Exercise can help you lose weight and control diabetes. Physical activity improves insulin sensitivity, meaning you won't need as much to handle the glucose in your bloodstream that comes from eating.

Exercise helps you build fat-burning muscle. A new study by researchers at Wake Forest University suggests combining weight training with a low-calorie diet preserves lean muscle mass that steadily declines with age. It appears that it's never too late to reap the benefits of strength training. In another study, researchers from Purdue University put men and women (average age 61) through a simple workout program and found that they were able to lose fat and pounds, get stronger, and improve their blood sugar control. At the end of the 12-week plan, the subjects gained four pounds of lean muscle and lost four pounds of fat.

When Exercise Backfires

Working out can add pounds instead of subtract them in certain cases.

Exercise can also cause you to put on weight if you aren't careful. Research has found that workouts do make you hungrier. You may feel that you deserve to eat junk food as a reward for all your hard work. But a study in the journal *Obesity Reviews* determined that people tend to overestimate the effect of exercise and overcompensate by eating a lot more calories than they burned during a workout. The solution is to practice mindful eating, get on an exercise plan, and use smoothies to refuel without overdoing the calories.

The Workout That Doesn't Feel Like Working Out

If you don't like going to a gym for whatever reason, the 7-Day Smoothie Diet fitness plan is custom made for you. You can do it at home or at work or just about anywhere you happen to be. It builds mini workouts into your normal daily activities. That way, you don't have to make time to exercise, which is hard to do as busy as we are these days. You don't even have to change into workout clothes if you don't want to. You don't have to go to a gym, because there's no special gear required. You already own the equipment you need: Your body is your gym. That means there's never an excuse not to do something that can improve your life. That's the premise behind the fitness plan here: Look for ways to turn nonproductive time into opportunities to get your body moving!

Here's a basic outline of possibilities. Use it as a guide and customize it according to your daily activities.

IN YOUR BEDROOM:

The Wake-Up Five

Start your morning off right with these five dynamic moves as soon as you get out of bed to get the blood flowing and the cobwebs out.

1. Hug

Stand with your feet hip-width apart and your arms out to your sides, palms forward, so your body and arms form a T. Quickly

give yourself a big bear hug, wrapping your arms around your torso. Then swing your arms out to the starting position. Do 20 times.

2. Reach

Stand with your feet hip-width apart. Spread your fingertips wide and reach your arms overhead as high as you can. Pause for two seconds and feel your body elongate. Then bend your elbows and lower your arms to chest level while keeping your elbows spread out to the sides. Do 6 times.

3. Power Lunge

Adapted from a popular runner's stretch, this lunge becomes a full-body movement with the addition of a sky reach. Start by standing straight with feet hip-width apart. Take a giant step forward with your left foot, keeping your right foot in place. Bend your left knee until your thigh and lower leg form a right angle. Your left knee should be directly over your ankle and your back leg should be straight, your heel raised and your weight on the ball of your right foot. Now raise your arms straight up toward the ceiling, palms facing, fingers spread. Hold this position for three breaths, then step back and repeat the Power Lunge with your right foot forward.

4. Cat/Cow

A classic yoga pose to stretch the lower back and relieve tension in the shoulders. With hands on the floor directly under your shoulders, and knees directly under your hips, slowly round your back (cat) while pushing your head down.

Hold for a breath, then lift your head as you lower your belly toward the floor (cow). That's one repetition; do 4.

5. Bear Walk

This is a safe "animal move" that engages your entire body, getting the blood pumping. Get on your hands and knees on the carpet or a mat on the floor. Your hands should be directly under your shoulders, your knees directly under your hips. Now press into the floor with your toes to lift your knees off the floor an inch or two. Your upper and lower legs should form right angles. This is the starting position. Now, simultaneously lift and move your right hand and left foot forward about two inches. Press both into the floor, and move your left hand and right foot forward the same distance. Keep your core braced as if expecting someone to punch you in the stomach. Continue "bear walking" forward about five steps, then reverse the movement and bear walk backward five steps.

IN THE KITCHEN: Stretch and Strengthen

You spend a lot of time in your kitchen waiting for things to boil or broil or bake, right? Well, use that waiting-around time to get moving! Here are some ways. You can do all of these moves or just a few, but try to get them all in during the various times you spend in the kitchen over the course of the day.

1. High/Low Cabinet Reach

While you are putting groceries away or moving dishes from

the dishwasher to the cabinets, reach up, elongating your spine and flexing your shoulders to reach the high cabinet shelves. When you need to hit the low cabinets, don't bend at the waist with straight legs. Instead, get your whole body into the act by bending your knees or lunging to get low.

2. Counter Push-up

The kitchen offers a great opportunity to do a little upper-body strength work on the sturdy kitchen counters or maybe the island. Do hands-elevated push-ups to strengthen and tone your chest and arm muscles. Place your hands shoulder-width apart on the edge of the counter or island and take two or three steps backward away from the counter. Straighten your arms. Now, keeping your abs tight and your back straight, bend your arms to slowly lower your chest to the counter. Keep your elbows close to your sides; don't splay them out like a bird's wings. When your chest touches the counter, slowly press your body up until your arms are once again straight. Repeat. Do up to 12 repetitions.

3. Can-o-Beans Curl

Tone your arms without dumbbells. Use cans of beans or soup for your weights. Hold two cans of equal weight in your hands at your sides, palms facing up. Keeping your upper arms against your sides, bend your elbows to slowly raise the cans to your shoulders. Pause, then ever so slowly lower the weights back to a straight-arm position. Try to take 7 to 10 seconds during the lowering of the weights. You'll feel it working. Try for 10 to 12 repetitions. If you have time, do more sets.

4. Triceps Press-Back with Soup Can

Those bean-can curls work your biceps. Now you need to work the smaller muscles on the backs of your upper arms called the triceps. Grab one soup can in your right hand. Take a small step forward with your left foot and bend that knee slightly. Bend forward toward that knee and place your left hand on that knee. Now, press your upper right arm against your torso and bend your arm to a 90-degree angle. Keep your wrist straight, holding the can so it is close to your body. This is the starting position. Now, without moving your upper arm, extend your arm straight, pressing the soup can behind you. You should feel the tension in the back of your arm. Slowly return to the starting position and repeat. Do 10 to 12 repetitions, then repeat the press-back with the can in your left hand and your right foot forward.

5. Wall Sit

This is a terrific lower-body exercise that you can do anywhere, any time, not only when in the kitchen. All you need is a wall. Stand straight with your back pressing against a wall and take one step forward with both feet. Now bend your knees to "sit" in an imaginary chair. Lower your body until your thighs are parallel with the floor. If that's too hard, stop when your thighs are at a 45-degree angle to the floor. Make sure your knees don't travel forward over your toes. Pressing your back into the wall for support, hold this position for as long as you can. Try for 30 seconds before standing. If that's easy, work your way toward 60-second holds before rising.

AT WORK OR DOING CHORES:
The Afternoon Energizer

Use your time at work or while running errands or doing chores to engage your entire body. Here are some ideas you may have heard of. But are you doing them?

- Park in the farthest spot away from the door of your destination to force yourself to do a little walk. Inside, take the stairs instead of the elevator. Doing this every day adds up.
- Whenever the phone rings or someone comes to visit, stand up. Standing will energize you, burn slightly more calories than sitting does, and make your phone voice sound richer.
- Drop the phone. Instead of calling or texting a colleague or neighbor, take a walk to visit.
- After lunch, go to the stairwell and do a series of stair climbs. Briskly walk up, then slowly walk back down. To add resistance, take two stairs at a time going up.
- Need to pee? Use the upstairs bathroom to force yourself to walk more.

1. **Chair Sit and Stand.** Get the blood flowing and strengthen your legs by standing in front of a chair and slowly lowering your body until your butt hits the seat cushion. Don't plop down, but keep the tension on. As soon as you touch, press your feet into the floor to slowly stand straight up. Repeat 20 sit-and-stands three times a day.

2. **Door Chest Stretch.** Stand in the middle of a standard doorway. Bend your arms to raise them so you can place your elbows and each side of your arms against the

doorframe. Your upper arms should be about parallel with the floor, your forearms pointing toward the ceiling. Carefully lean forward through the doorway until you can feel the stretch in your chest. Hold for three seconds, release, and repeat at least 3 times. Do this several times a day to improve your posture and stretch your rounded back muscles.

3. **Pickups or Lunges.** Throw a few paper clips on the floor of the office. Pick them up by lunging forward or bending your knees and rising up. If you are vacuuming the rug, with each push forward do an alternating forward lunge.

4. **Farmer's Carry.** Improve grip strength, get your heart rate up, and burn extra calories with this simple, safe exercise. Hold something heavy of equal weight in each hand by its handle. Use gallon jugs of water, encyclopedias, buckets filled with water or stones, canvas bags of groceries, whatever's convenient. Hold the weights with arms held straight down and simply walk. Technique tips:

- Keep your shoulders tight to protect the joints.
- Think of these walks as walking planks. Keep your core engaged. Tuck your chin to keep your head, ears, and back aligned over your pelvis as you walk.
- Take short steps to ensure a more stable base.
- Walk 10 steps, turn around and walk back. Rest. Do two more sets.

Dress Down, Drop Pounds

If your dress code allows, wear jeans to work. A study by the American Council on Exercise found that casual clothing, as opposed to traditional business attire, could increase physical activity levels in one's daily routine. Participants in the study took an additional 491 steps and burned 25 more calories on days they wore denim as opposed to when wearing traditional work attire. That may not sound like much, but one casual Friday a week could slash 6,250 calories over the course of the year—enough to offset the average annual weight gain (0.4 to 1.8 pounds) experienced by most Americans.

AFTER DINNER:

The 10-Minute Walking Secret

Walking after a meal aids digestion and makes you feel better. You don't need a study to prove that to you. But do you do it regularly? Would you do it if you knew that it could reduce your cravings for dessert and even help you lose weight?

Check out this recent study on people with type 2 diabetes from researchers in New Zealand. Scientists from the University of Otago recruited 41 people with diabetes, ages 18 to 75, and randomly placed them into one of two groups. One group took a 30-minute walk each day. The other group took a 10-minute walk each day after every meal, totaling 30 minutes. All the participants wore exercise monitors and filled out detailed food diaries. Their blood sugar levels were regularly monitored. The results of the 14-day test, reported in the journal *Diabetologia*: The researchers found that when people walked for 10 minutes after a meal, their blood sugar levels were on average 12 percent lower than the glucose levels of people who walked for 30 minutes once a day. Even more interesting, blood sugar levels of the 10-minute walkers were 22 percent lower than the 30-minute walkers' in the evening after dinner. The researchers believe that the greater reduction is due to the fact that the evening meal typically contained a larger percentage of carbohydrates than the other two meals, and people tend to be more sedentary in the evening.

What does this mean for you? Consider this: Walking after a meal acts like insulin. By using your muscles and elevating your heart rate, your body more efficiently clears glucose from your bloodstream and moves it into your muscles. So by following the 7-Day Smoothie Diet plan and going for a walk after dinner each night, you may help keep blood sugar from turning into body fat, and you automatically avoid the cravings for a sweet dessert that can result from swings in blood sugar levels.

Go for a 10- to 20-minute walk within a half hour after dinner, even if you must leave the dirty dishes in the sink! Do it every evening for seven days, and it will become an enjoyable ritual you won't want to miss.

WHILE WATCHING TV: Focus on Your Core

You're just sitting there on the couch. Why not burn a few more calories and strengthen your body while watching the news or binging on your favorite Netflix show?

Hate doing core exercises? Do them while your mind is occupied with *Wheel of Fortune* and they'll be done before final spin. Try these easy moves during the commercials:

1. Superwoman to Aqua Man. This is a fun exercise that's great for lower-back strength and flexibility. Lie facedown on the floor with your arms outstretched straight over your head, palms on the floor, and toes pointed behind you. Take a breath and lift your straight arms and straight legs off the floor as high as you can without causing pain. Hold that position for two seconds, then exhale and relax back to the floor. Repeat four more times. On your fifth Superwoman move, paddle your outstretched arms and legs up and down as if you were splashing in a pool: right arm and left leg up, left arm and right leg down, and alternate for as long as you can. That's Aqua Man.

2. Plank. Get into the top of a push-up position with your arms straight, hands directly under your shoulders. You'll be on the balls of your feet, and your back should be straight from your head to your heels. Engage your abs and lower back to keep your hips from sinking. Gaze at the floor. Try to hold this position for 30 seconds, working up to a full minute over time. If this becomes too easy, try the plank on your forearms. Simply bend your arms and support yourself on your forearms, elbows directly under your shoulders.

3. Side Plank. This one you can do while watching TV. Lie on your right side with your legs straight. Prop yourself up with your right forearm so your body forms a diagonal line. Rest your left hand on your hip. Engage your abs and hold for 30 seconds. Be sure your hips don't sag to the floor. If you can't make it to 30 seconds, hold for 5 to 10 seconds and rest for 5; continue for 30 seconds. Work up to 60 seconds. Repeat on your left side.

4. **Hip Raise.** Lie on your back on the floor and bend your knees so your heels are three to five inches from your buttocks or as close to that as you can. Place your arms flat on the floor at a 45-degree angle to your body, palms down. Press your feet into the floor to lift your hips until your thighs, hips, and chest form a straight line. Pause in this up position for two seconds, squeezing your buttocks and engaging your abs, then slowly lower yourself to the floor and repeat 4 more times.

Want to do some more? Add in a chair sit, air squat (like a chair sit without the chair), bear crawl, or power lunge.

BEFORE BED:

The Yoga Sequence

A nighttime stretching and strengthening routine will prepare your body for more restful sleep. The sequence below will raise your body temperature slightly. That's good. But the last two poses in the sequence will start to bring your core temperature down, which encourages sleep.

1. **Cat/Cow**

Repeat the pose you did in the morning to relieve the day's pent-up tension in your lower back and shoulders. With hands on floor directly under your shoulders and knees directly under your hips, slowly round your back (cat) while pushing your head down. Hold for a breath, then lift your head as you lower your belly toward the floor (cow). That's a single rep; do 4.

2. Child's Pose

Kneel on the floor with your knees a bit wider than hip-width apart and your big toes touching behind you. Now bend forward and reach your arms on the floor over your head, palms down. Try to get your forehead down to the floor. Inhale deeply and exhale for 5 breaths.

3. Sphinx

Lie facedown on the floor with your toes pointed behind you. Bend your elbows and bring your hands, palms down, next to your shoulders as in the down push-up position. Slowly press your hands into the floor to raise your head and shoulders off the floor while keeping your hips pressed into the floor. The movement is subtle. Don't arch your back too much. Hold the raised position for three breaths; lower and repeat twice more.

4. Reclining Bound Angle

Lie back on pillows supporting your upper and middle back. Rest your head on a folded blanket. Press the soles of your feet together and let your knees fall open to both sides, opening your hips. Pull your shoulder blades inward slightly, and allow your arms to rest at your sides, palms facing up. Breathe deeply, close your eyes, and relax for a minute or two. If you feel strain in the hips or groin, place pillows or yoga blocks under your knees.

5. Savasana

From the Reclining Bound Angle position (above), straighten your legs, and remove the pillows from under your back and head. Your feet should be hip-width apart. Allow your feet to fall toward the sides as they may. Your arms should be relaxed at your sides, palms up. Relax and breathe deeply. Stay in this meditative position until you are just about to fall asleep. And it's okay if you do.

Bathroom Fitness

Strengthen your ankles while brushing your teeth.

Stand on one foot on a pillow with your other foot raised behind you. The unstable surface will engage the small muscles supporting that ankle to keep you balanced. Brushing your teeth with your nondominant hand makes balancing harder and challenges your brain as well. Halfway through brushing, stand on the other foot.

Extra Effort: The Daily Burn

Want to kick your metabolism into overdrive? Then add one of these two extra-effort workouts every day during your 7-Day Smoothie Diet. (Or replace one of these new workouts for one of your daily "move more" sessions.)

A. One 15-minute High Intensity Interval Training (HIIT) exercise routine.

Or

B. Body weight exercise circuit called the Fire Drill.

Both will get your heart pounding, improve your endurance, and challenge your strength. But don't fear. You can do them!

Which one you do on any given day is up to you. When you do the workout is up to you, too. Early morning is a great opportunity to get it out of the way, but if that doesn't work for you, then do it at midmorning, at lunchtime, or in the afternoon. Just get A or B done before dinnertime.

If you want to lose weight, get lean and fit, High Intensity Interval Training, or HIIT for short, is your ticket. No exercise routine is quite as effective as when you push yourself to a higher level of effort. How do you know if you are exercising intensely enough? Easy. Here's the test: If you can carry on a normal conversation while exercising, you're not working hard enough. If you're huffing and puffing and find it hard to speak in full sentences, you're exercising hard enough.

Pick your favorite form of exercise for your HIIT workout: Walking, running, bicycling, working out on an elliptical machine or stair stepper. Your choice. You can choreograph a HIIT workout for almost any type of exercise. The key is to intersperse segments of rigorous (fast) effort with periods of "active rest" done at a slower pace and a much lower physical intensity.

EXTRA EFFORT A: The HIIT Workout

Here's one way to go for a walk or ride, HIIT-style:

> **2-minute warm-up at a slow pace**

> **1-minute medium pace**

> **30 seconds fast pace (hard to speak in sentences)**

> 1-minute active resting pace (you're moving, but a lot slower and able to speak comfortably)
> 30 seconds fast pace
> 1 minute active resting pace
> 1 minute fast pace
> 1 minute active resting pace
> 30 seconds fast pace
> 30 seconds active resting pace
> 30 seconds fast pace
> 30 seconds active resting pace
> 1 minute fast pace
> 1 minute active resting pace
> 2 minutes cool-down at slow pace

If you do the HIIT workout one day, do the Fire Drill the next.

EXTRA EFFORT B:
The Fire Drill

For days when you don't have much time, do this superquick heart-pumping strength workout, which takes less than 7 minutes. If you find a particular exercise too challenging, try its easier option.

Warm-up: March in place with knees raised high. Punch your hands, in alternating fashion, into the sky for about a minute.

1. **Mountain Climber.** Start in a plank position with your arms straight, hands directly under your shoulders. Keep your abs pulled in and your body straight. Pull your right knee to your chest. Quickly switch and pull the left knee to your chest

as you straighten the right. That's one repetition. Continue to alternate knees using a running motion. **Do 20 repetitions.** [Easier: Hands-Elevated Mountain Climber. Place your hands on the edge of a tub or the arm of a sofa with arms straight. Engage your abs. Pump your legs in a running motion.]

Active Rest. Stand with arms outstretched so your body forms a T. Roll your arms forward in small circles increasing in size to large circles. After 10 circles, reverse the direction for 10.

2. **Jump Squat.** Stand with feet shoulder-width apart, arms at your sides. Bend your knees to squat as if sitting in a chair until your thighs are parallel with the floor. Then press your feet into the floor and jump explosively into the air, swinging your arms up to help propel you. As soon as your feet touch down, lower into another squat and repeat. **Do 10 reps.** [Easier: Air Squat. If your knees bother you, don't jump. Just air squat. When your thighs reach a position where they are parallel with the floor, press your feet into the floor and slowly rise.]

Rest. Walk around and shake out your legs for up to a minute.

3. **On-Knees Push-Up.** Get on all fours with knees directly under your hips and your hands directly under your shoulders. Cross your feet, one over the other, behind you. Keeping your core engaged, bend your arms to lower your torso toward the floor. When your chin is an inch above the

floor, straighten your arms. That's one rep. Do 10 reps.
[Easier: Wall Push-Up. If you cannot do On-Knees Push-ups, work up to them by doing the Wall Push-Up. Stand facing a wall. Place your hands on the wall at shoulder-height with arms straight. You'll need to step back a few feet from the wall. Engage your abs and bend your arms to lower your body toward the wall. When your head nears the wall, straighten your arms. That's one rep. Do 10 reps.]

Rest for 30 seconds to a minute.

4. **Elbow to Knee.** Stand straight with feet shoulder width apart and arms spread out to your sides forming a T. Raise your right knee and angle it across your body while simultaneously bending your left elbow and bringing it to meet your right knee. Return to start, then raise your left knee to meet your right elbow. That's one repetition. Keep alternating sides for 10 total reps.
[Easier: Do another 10 high-knee marches.]

No Rest.

5. **Bear Walk.** Get on your hands and knees on the carpet. Your hands should be directly under your shoulders, your knees directly under your hips. Now press into the floor with your toes to lift your knees off the floor an inch or two. Your upper and lower legs should form right angles. This is the starting position. Now, simultaneously lift and move your right hand and left foot forward about two inches. Press both into the floor, and move your left hand and right foot forward the

same distance. Keep your core braced as if expecting someone to punch you in the stomach. Continue "bear walking" forward for 10 feet.

FINISHER (optional):
Another set of Jump Squats. If you have enough energy to do more after the Bear Walk, try this finisher: Go right into another set of 10 Jump Squats.

You're done!
Remember: If you do the Fire Drill one day, do the HIIT workout the next, and so on.

Do The 10-Minute "Mountain" Climb

To kick your fat-burners into high gear—and get a great aerobic workout in a short time—find a set of stairs and climb!

The standard staircase grade is steep, forcing you to exert much more leg strength to lift your body weight. As a result, each step up you take increases the metabolic intensity of even slow walking. You can easily boost your leg strength, elevate your heart rate, and increase your endurance by mixing in an occasional "mountain climb." Go to a high school athletic field's grandstand or even the emergency stairwell of a school or your place of work. After a walking warm-up on flat ground, hit the stairs. Climb at a slow to moderate pace. (You don't have to go fast.) Turn around at the top and walk down. Repeat for 10 minutes.

CHAPTER

8

Your Day-to-Day Checklist

MOST PEOPLE START feeling the results of the 7-Day Smoothie Diet within the first two days. By eliminating added sugars and starchy processed foods from your diet and replacing them with nutritious, satisfying smoothies and extra-filling meals, you'll automatically reduce your calories and avoid binge-triggering cravings. By the end of the week, your pants may feel a little looser; the scale will likely show a few pounds gone, seven or maybe more! But that's not your end-all goal. It's just the beginning—the beginning of a life of healthy, mindful eating and greater respect for your miraculous body.

The 7-Day Smoothie Diet is designed to introduce you to a smarter, healthier way of living. You'll see and feel quick results, which will prove to you what you're capable of doing in short order. And it will motivate you to continue along the path of taking better care of your body so you will look better, feel better, and enjoy the powerful sense of control you have over your health destiny.

But the 7-Day Smoothie Diet is not a walk in the park—although a walk in the park is a fine idea for after dinner! No, anything worthwhile that you'd like to accomplish takes some discipline. And the 7-Day Smoothie Diet is likely to be more intense than other weight-loss programs you may have tried. That's why it's only seven days long. You can do anything for seven days. And we're asking you to be disciplined for one week so that you can fully experience and appreciate the lifestyle changes this plan introduces.

After a week on this plan, you will be convinced that swapping out those carb-heavy, processed foods loaded with sugar and dense calories devoid of nutrients in favor of smoothies and other clean foods leads to a better life. You will become a mindful eater who understands that there are choices to make every day. One choice will make you look and feel better. The other will make you heavier, less energetic, and unhealthy.

You will make the right choice when you experience the difference healthier eating makes. To experience that, you need to be disciplined. Make it easier on yourself by having a master plan. It's as simple as making up a to-do list and checking off each box as you complete each required task. Not only does it keep you accountable, it makes it easier to remember what to do. You're not relying on memory. What's more? It's motivating. If you've ever used to-do lists, you know what we mean. Doesn't it feel great at the end of the day when you've accomplished everything you've set out to do?

So, here's your to-do list for the next seven days. Follow our suggestions or adapt this list to your preferences. But use it. Check off each important piece of the plan as you complete it and watch the pounds melt away. At the end of the week, embark on your new life of more mindful eating and exercise. You can return to this seven-day plan whenever you feel you need a boost to get back on track or you have a special event for which you want to feel and look your best. Here's what the 7-Day Smoothie Diet plan looks like, day by day.

Day 1

____ Do the Wake-Up Five exercises as soon as you get out of bed to jumpstart your day.

____ Drink your tall glass of lemon water.

____ Make your morning smoothie and sip it as you think about the day before you. Plan your afternoon smoothie. Do you need to make it at home to take to work?
Suggestions for ...
Morning: The Blueberry Granola Bowl (page 53)
Afternoon: The Coffee Break Smoothie (page 54)

____ **Do you need coffee?** Have a small cup (6 ounces) black or with a little half-and-half, but no sugar. If you must have a little sweetener, use stevia. But ideally get away from sweeteners in your coffee. Or, better yet, have a cup of tea. Black, white, green, or herbal tea is fine. No sweeteners.

____ Get moving! Are you working some extra movement exercises into your morning? Review Chapter 7 for suggestions.

____ Midmorning: Use a Cravings Crusher technique (Chapter 6) if you have any hunger pangs. Drink more water or have a cup of fat-blocking tea.

____ **Lunch extra-filling food suggestion:** Avocado Black Bean Salad (page 112). Drink lemon water, unsweetened iced tea, or hot tea.

____ Have your afternoon Coffee Break Smoothie whenever you feel you start to feel a little hungry.

____ Get moving! Walk up and down a flight of stairs.

____ Optional Extra Effort A or B.

____ **Dinner suggestion:** Portobello Turkey Burger and Bruschetta with Strawberry Pecan Salad (page 126).

____ Walk for 10 minutes, preferably outside, at a slow to moderate pace.

____ Get moving! Are you working some extra movement exercises into your evening? Do something active while watching TV.

____ Before bed: Do the Yoga Calm sequence to prepare your body for sleep.

Congratulations! Doesn't a structured day of healthy living feel great?

Day 2

____ Wake-Up Five exercises.

____ Drink your glass of lemon water.

____ **Morning smoothie suggestion:** Chocolate Peanut Butter Power House Smoothie (page 50).

____ Get moving!

____ Midmorning: Have a fat-blocking cup of tea.

____ **Lunch suggestion:** Broth-based soup, Tuna Salad Wrap (page 113).

____ **Afternoon smoothie suggestion:** Fruit Loopers Smoothie (page 57).

____ Get moving!

____ Optional Extra Effort A or B.

____ **Dinner suggestion:** Quickie Chili (page 122). Drink lemon water, unsweetened iced tea, or hot tea.

____ After-dinner walk (10 minutes).

____ Get moving!

____ Yoga Calm sequence.

Day 3

____ Wake-Up Five exercises.

____ Drink your glass of lemon water.

____ **Morning smoothie suggestion:** Walnut Mint Chip (page 51).

____ Get moving!

____ Midmorning: Have a fat-blocking cup of tea.

____ Lunch suggestion: Vegetable Omelet (page 113). Drink lemon water, unsweetened iced tea, or hot tea.

____ **Afternoon smoothie suggestion:** Apple Flax Smoothie (page 153).

____ Get moving!

____ Optional Extra Effort A or B.

____ **Dinner suggestion:** Pan-Seared Salmon with Basil, side dish of broccoli or asparagus (page 124).

____ After-dinner walk (10 minutes).

____ Get moving!

____ Yoga Calm sequence.

Day 4

____ Wake-Up Five exercises.

____ Drink your glass of lemon water.

____ **Morning smoothie suggestion:** Mega Greens Smoothie, page 50, (make enough for afternoon, too).

____ Get moving!.

____ Midmorning: Have a fat-blocking cup of tea.

____ Lunch suggestion: Chicken Salad with Pistachios (page 115). Drink lemon water, unsweetened iced tea, or hot tea.

____ **Afternoon smoothie suggestion:** leftover Mega Greens Smoothie.

____ Get moving!

____ Optional Extra Effort A or B.

____ **Dinner suggestion:** Vegan Red Lentil Soup (page 125). Drink lemon water, unsweetened iced tea, or hot tea.

____ After-dinner walk (10 minutes).

____ Get moving!

____ Yoga Calm sequence.

Day 5

____ Wake-Up Five exercises.

____ Drink your glass of lemon water.

____ **Morning smoothie suggestion:** Acai Almond Smoothie Bowl (page 139).

____ Get moving!

____ Midmorning: Have a fat-blocking cup of tea.

____ **Lunch suggestion:** Make-Ahead Quinoa and Roasted Broccoli Bowl (page 114). Drink lemon water, unsweetened iced tea, or hot tea.

____ **Afternoon smoothie suggestion:** Sweet Baby Kale (page 135).

____ Get moving!

____ Optional Extra Effort A or B.

____ **Dinner suggestion:** Turkey Meat Loaf (page 123) with any vegetable side you'd like.

____ After-dinner walk (10 minutes).

____ Get moving!

____ Yoga Calm sequence.

Day 6

____ Wake-Up Five exercises.

____ Drink your glass of lemon water.

____ **Morning smoothie suggestion:** PB & JP Smoothie (page 49).

____ Get moving!

____ Midmorning: Have a fat-blocking cup of tea.

____ **Lunch suggestion:** Mediterranean Hummus Wrap (page 112). Drink lemon water, unsweetened iced tea, or hot tea.

____ **Afternoon smoothie suggestion:** Green Hornet Smoothie (page 136).

____ Get moving!

____ Optional Extra Effort A or B.

____ **Dinner suggestion:** Leftover Turkey Meat Loaf.

____ After-dinner walk (10 minutes).

____ Get moving!

____ Yoga Calm sequence.

Day 7

____ Wake-Up Five exercises.

____ Drink your glass of lemon water.

____ **Morning smoothie:** Strawberry Olive Oil Smoothie (page 135).

____ Get moving!

____ **Midmorning:** Have a fat-blocking cup of tea.

____ Lunch suggestion: Minestrone Soup (page 116) with a side salad. Drink lemon water, unsweetened iced tea, or hot tea.

____ **Afternoon smoothie suggestion:** Carrot with a Kick (page 56).

____ Get moving!

____ Optional Extra Effort A or B.

____ **Dinner suggestion:** Sheet Pan Roasted Vegetables with Chicken (page 122). Drink lemon water, unsweetened iced tea, or hot tea.

____ After-dinner walk (10 minutes).

____ Get moving!

____ Yoga Calm sequence.

CHAPTER

9

The Smoothie Diet Lunch and Dinner Recipes

How to prepare the gourmet-quality lunches and dinners you'll enjoy during the 7-Day Smoothie Diet

HERE ARE SOME terrific options for homemade lunches to choose from during your diet week. You don't have to eat them in this order. In fact, if you like one in particular, you can have it more than once during the week. And if you prefer to eat out for lunch, just make sure that you have a protein-rich salad or a broth soup and a protein-rich sandwich. Try to avoid the second slice of bread.

Lunches

Avocado Black Bean Salad

2 cups romaine lettuce hearts, chopped
1 medium avocado, chopped into bite-size pieces
1 medium tomato, chopped into bite-size pieces
½ cup canned black beans, rinsed and drained
2 Tbsp. diced green onion
1 Tbsp. diced fresh cilantro
1 Tbsp. olive oil
2 tsp. lime juice
1 tsp. lime zest
¼ tsp. salt
½ tsp. ground black pepper

- Toss the lettuce, avocado, tomato, beans, green onion, and cilantro in a large salad bowl.
- In a small bowl, stir together the olive oil, lime juice, lime zest, salt, and pepper. Pour over the salad, and toss to coat.

Makes 2 servings.

Per serving: 247 calories, 17 g fat, 20 g carbohydrates, 9 g fiber, 6 g protein

Mediterranean Hummus Wrap

¼ cup roasted red pepper hummus
1 100% whole-wheat wrap (9-inch diameter)
2 zucchini strips, sliced thinly lengthwise
1 Tbsp. kalamata olives, pitted
¼ cup shredded carrots
4 thinly sliced tomato slices
½ cup shredded romaine lettuce
¼ cup feta cheese

- Spread the hummus on the bottom half of the wrap.

- Layer the zucchini strips, olives, carrots, tomatoes, and lettuce in the center of the wrap. Crumble the feta cheese on top of the veggies.
- Roll the wrap from the hummus side, fold the sides in, and continue to roll the sandwich into a pocket.
- Cut the wrap in half on an angle.

Makes one serving.

Per serving: 372 calories, 17 g fat, 40 g carbohydrates, 8 g fiber, 17 g protein

---

Tuna Salad Wrap

1 can (or foil pouch) low-sodium, chunk white tuna in spring water
¼ cup minced onion
1 celery stalk, chopped
1 tsp. lemon juice
1 Tbsp. olive oil
1 Tbsp. chopped fresh parsley
¼ cup Dijon mustard
½ tsp. salt (or use No Salt or Nu-Salt)
½ tsp. pepper
2 whole-wheat tortillas

- Mix all the ingredients except the tortillas in a bowl.
- Spoon the mixture onto the tortilla and wrap. Whole-grain bread may be substituted for the tortilla to make a sandwich.

Makes 2 servings.

Per serving: 258 calories, 26 g fat, 29 g carbohydrate, 4 g fiber, 18 g protein

---

Vegetable Omelet

2 large eggs
1 Tbsp. flat-leaf parsley, chopped
Dash of reduced-sodium soy sauce
2 tsp. olive oil
½ cup baby spinach
1½ Tbsp. broccoli florets, chopped

2 asparagus spears, chopped
½ tsp. minced garlic
Dash ground black pepper

- Beat the eggs, parsley, and soy sauce in a bowl.
- Coat a large skillet with olive oil. Add the spinach, broccoli, asparagus, garlic, and pepper to the skillet and cook over medium heat for 5 minutes.
- Pour the egg mixture over the vegetables. Stir, and then let it sit for 1 minute. Stir again until the eggs are firm. Let sit another minute. Fold the omelet and remove to a plate.

Makes 1 serving.

Per serving: 262 calories, 17 g fat, 9 g carbohydrates, 3 g fiber, 19 g protein.

Make-Ahead Quinoa and Roasted Broccoli Bowl

1 lb. broccoli, cut into florets
1 Tbsp. extra-virgin olive oil
Salt and pepper to taste
1 cup uncooked red quinoa, rinsed and drained
1 cup seedless grapes, halved
1 can (16 oz.) chickpeas, rinsed and drained
1 avocado, chopped
4 oz. goat cheese, crumbled
½ cup sliced almonds

For dressing:
½ cup extra-virgin olive oil
1 Tbsp. Dijon mustard
2 Tbsp. local honey
2 Tbsp. lemon juice
½ tsp. sea salt
Black pepper to taste

- Preheat oven to 425°F. Place the broccoli florets in a rimmed baking dish and toss with 1 tablespoon of olive oil. Sprinkle with salt and pepper. Roast the broccoli for 25 minutes or until crisp and tender.

- Combine the quinoa and two cups of water in a saucepan. Bring to a boil. Lower the heat to simmer; cover and simmer for 15 minutes, until water is absorbed.
- Make the salad dressing by whisking together all the dressing ingredients.
- Assemble each bowl by adding a quarter of the quinoa, broccoli, grapes, and chickpeas. Slice the avocado and divide among the four bowls. Crumble the goat cheese on top and sprinkle with the sliced almonds. Drizzle the dressing on top and serve.

Makes 4 servings.
Per serving (with dressing): 862 calories, 54 g fat, 77 g carbohydrates, 16 g fiber, 24 g protein

---

Chicken Salad with Pistachios

2 cups carrots, peeled and cut into slices
1 Tbsp. brown sugar
2 Tbsp. extra-virgin olive oil
½ tsp. salt
½ tsp. freshly ground black pepper
2 boneless, skinless chicken breast halves (6 oz. each), cut crosswise in thin slices
4 Tbsp. snipped fresh chives or sliced scallion greens
1 Tbsp. cider vinegar
1 tsp. apple cider vinegar
1 medium shallot, thinly sliced
2 cups arugula
1 bunch watercress, tough stems removed
1½ cups red seedless grapes, halved
2 Tbsp. unsalted shelled pistachios, chopped

- Preheat the oven to 425°F. Coat an 11" x 9" baking pan and a rimmed baking sheet with olive oil cooking spray.
- Place the carrots in the prepared baking pan. Sprinkle with the sugar, 1 teaspoon of the olive oil, and a pinch each of the salt and pepper. Toss to coat well. Roast, stirring several times, for 25 minutes, until the carrots are tender and lightly golden at the edges.

- About 5 minutes before the carrots are done, place the chicken in a mound on the prepared baking sheet. Drizzle with 1 teaspoon of the oil, and sprinkle with 2 tablespoons of the chives and a pinch each of the salt and pepper. Toss to mix. Arrange in a single layer. Roast, turning once, for 5 to 7 minutes, until cooked through. Remove carrots and chicken from the oven and let them cool a few minutes.

- In a salad bowl, mix the vinegar, shallot, remaining oil, 2 tablespoons chives, and ¼ teaspoon each salt and pepper. Let stand 5 minutes or more to blend the flavors.

- Add the arugula, watercress, and grapes to the dressing and toss to mix well. Spread out on a platter. Top with the carrots, the chicken and any juices, and sprinkle with the pistachios. Serve warm.

Makes 4 servings.

Per serving: 307 calories, 10 fat, 32 g carbohydrates, 4.5 g fiber, 23 g protein

---

Minestrone Soup

1 lb. sweet Italian chicken sausage, cut into 1-in. chunks
2 cloves garlic, minced
1 medium yellow onion, chopped
2 ribs celery, chopped
1 carrot, chopped
4 cups water
1 can (16 oz.) reduced-sodium chicken broth
1 can (6 oz.) tomato paste
1 can (14 oz.) kidney beans, rinsed and drained
1 can (15 oz.) corn, drained
3 Tbsp. dried pearl barley
Salt and ground black pepper
1 cup ditalini pasta
4 Tbsp. grated Parmesan cheese

- Heat a large pot over medium heat. Add the sausage and cook for about 10 minutes, stirring occasionally. Remove the sausage from the pot and pour off the liquid and fat.

- Add the garlic, onion, celery, and carrots, and return the pot to the stove. Cook for about 3 minutes until the vegetables are soft.

- Add the water, broth, tomato paste, kidney beans, corn, and barley. Add the salt and pepper. Raise heat and bring to a boil, then reduce heat to low and simmer for 20 minutes.
- Add the pasta and stir. Cook until done, about 10 minutes. Sprinkle with Parmesan cheese.

Makes 4 servings.

Per 2 cup serving: 340 calories, 7 g fat, 47 g carbohydrates, 7 g fiber, 22 g protein

---

Cobb Salad

3 cups Boston bibb, red or green leaf lettuce, chopped
3 cups baby spinach, chopped
2 Tbsp. red wine vinegar
8 oz. turkey breast, sliced
1 avocado, cubed
1 cup canned cannellini beans, rinsed
1 large tomato, diced
2 cups English cucumber, chopped
2 Tbsp. bleu cheese, crumbled
2 hard-boiled eggs, diced

- Toss the lettuce and spinach in a bowl with the red wine vinegar.
- Plate the lettuce and arrange the remaining ingredients in strips over the top.

Makes 4 servings.

Per serving: 270 calories, 10.7 g fat, 15.7 g carbohydrates, 7.8 g fiber, 30 g protein

The Ultimate Salad

Recruit a rainbow coalition of nutritious vegetables and protein.

The best way to get your essential vitamins and antioxidants is straight from the source: a fresh salad full of greens and vegetables in a rainbow of colors. A study by the Louisiana State University School of Public Health found that people who eat a salad a day are more likely to get their recommended daily intake of many essential nutrients. There's also evidence that a salad a day may increase your lifespan. Salad day after day can quickly become unsatisfying unless you doctor it up a bit with new ingredients. Here's how to turn a salad into a memorable meal.

THE BASE:

Spinach and Red-leaf lettuce

■ One cup of spinach gives you 58 micrograms (mcg) of folate. According to a study in the journal *Stroke*, consuming at least 300 mcg of folate a day reduces your risk of having a stroke by 20 percent and decreases your risk of developing heart disease by 13 percent. Other studies have found that folate helps protect against both Alzheimer's disease and cancer. Four leaves of red-leaf lettuce contain 1,213 mcg of antioxidants, 96 mcg of vitamin K (which has been shown to maintain bone mass), and 1,172 mcg of the carotenoids lutein and zeaxanthin. The National Institutes of Health found that lutein and zeaxanthin can decrease your risk of developing macular degeneration by 43 percent.

Other nutrients: fiber, protein, vitamin A, vitamin B6, vitamin C, vitamin E, vitamin K, calcium, and potassium

---

THE CRUNCH:

Broccoli

■ You get 294 milligrams (mg) of potassium in just three spears. According to Mayo Clinic researchers, potassium counteracts the effects of sodium by dilating blood vessels and increasing the amount of sodium excreted in your urine, thus lowering blood pressure.

Other nutrients: calcium, fiber, vitamin, vitamin B6, vitamin C, vitamin K, folate, lutein, and zeaxanthin

---

THE FIBER:

Red kidney beans

■ A one-cup serving of red kidney beans gives you 6,630 disease-fighting antioxidants, plus a full 3 grams of fiber. According to the American Dietetic Association, dietary fiber lowers blood cholesterol levels and helps normalize blood glucose and insulin levels, decreasing the risk of cardiovascular disease, metabolic syndrome, and type 2 diabetes.

Other nutrients: protein and folate

THE COLORS:

Yellow bell peppers and carrots

■ Four strips of yellow bell pepper provide 48 mg of free-radical fighting vitamin C (free radicals are rogue molecules that can damage cells and lead to cancer). According to a study in the *Journal of the American College of Nutrition*, levels of C-reactive protein—a blood marker for inflammation linked to heart disease—can be decreased by 24 percent if you consume 500 mg of vitamin C a day. Plus, nutrition researchers from Arizona State University reported that vitamin C can help with weight loss by assisting in fat oxidation, or the body's ability to burn fat. Carrots are one of the richest sources of pro-vitamin A carotenoids, plant compounds that provide color and function as antioxidants. Just 1 cup of shredded carrots provides 2,279 mcg of beta-carotene and 4,623 IU of vitamin A. According to a study in the journal *Thorax*, beta-carotene can slow the age-related decline of lung power. Vitamin A has also been shown to improve vision and bone growth, help regulate the immune system, and decrease the risk of lung cancer.

Other nutrients: vitamin C, vitamin K, fiber, folate, vitamin B6, and potassium

THE VITAMIN D AND CALCIUM:

Swiss cheese

■ Four cubes of Swiss cheese provide 476 mg of calcium and 26 IU of vitamin D. In a 20-year study, British researchers determined that men who consume more than 67 IU of vitamin D and 190 mg of calcium a day have half the risk of stroke compared to men who consume less. Vitamin D has also been associated with a decrease in the risk of pancreatic, prostate, and testicular cancers. A study in the *Journal of the National Cancer Institute* found that men with higher blood levels of vitamin D had a 17 percent reduction in total cancer incidence and a 29 percent reduction in total cancer deaths.

Other nutrients: protein and vitamin B12

THE GOOD FATS:

Extra-virgin olive oil and balsamic vinegar

■ One tablespoon of olive oil delivers 10 grams of monounsaturated fat. Research shows that men with diets high in monounsaturated fat have higher testosterone levels than those whose diets don't. Antioxidant-rich balsamic vinegar can improve vascular function when ingested with a high-fat food like olive oil, which contributes to a reduction in the risk of heart disease.

Disease-fighting power: Adding olive oil to red, green, orange, or yellow fruits and vegetables increases the amount of heart-saving, cancer-fighting, vision-boosting, immune-repairing, bone-strengthening vitamins such as A, E, and K, as well as carotenoids.

Sunflower seeds and flaxseed

■ One tablespoon of sunflower seeds provides 8.35 mcg of selenium. Harvard researchers discovered that men with high levels of selenium have a 49 percent lower incidence of advanced prostate cancer than those with the lowest levels. One tablespoon of flaxseed will give you 2.3 grams of omega-3 fatty acids, which are linked to reduced risk of heart disease, Alzheimer's disease, and depression. They have also been shown to inhibit cancer-cell growth.

Other nutrients: vitamin E and fiber

Almonds

■ One tablespoon of almonds provides 2.2 grams of alpha-tocopherol, a type of vitamin E, which reduces the risk of Alzheimer's disease, according to a National Institute on Aging study. Another study showed that people who were clinically depressed had lower levels of alpha-tocopherol than their happy peers. Vitamin E also fights free-radical damage.

Other nutrients: monounsaturated fat, protein, and fiber

THE LYCOPENE:

Tomatoes

■ Four cherry tomatoes give you 1,748 mcg of the powerful antioxidant lycopene. A study in the *Journal of the National Cancer Institute* found that increasing dietary lycopene intake to 30 mg reduces oxidative DNA damage to prostate tissues and decreases PSA levels.

Other nutrients: vitamin A, vitamin C, vitamin K, fiber, and potassium

THE LEAN PROTEIN:

Chunk light tuna

■ Tuna, one of the best sources of protein, contains no trans fat, and a 3-oz. serving of chunk light tuna contains 11 mg of heart-healthy niacin, which has been shown to help lower cholesterol and help your body process fat. University of Rochester researchers determined that niacin raises HDL cholesterol (the good kind) and lowers triglycerides more than most statins alone.

Other nutrients: protein, selenium, and vitamin B12

Dinners

Sheet Pan–Roasted Vegetables with Chicken

6 Tbsp. balsamic vinegar
1½ Tbsp. Sriracha chili sauce
1½ Tbsp. local honey
1½ tsp. minced ginger
1½ tsp. minced garlic
½ tsp. black pepper
2½ lbs. boneless, skinless chicken breasts, cut into cubes
2 heads broccoli, cut into florets
2 orange or yellow bell peppers
1 red onion
½ head cauliflower, cut into florets

- Mix the vinegar, chili sauce, honey, ginger, garlic, and pepper in a bowl. Pour three quarters of the mixture into a large resealable plastic bag. Add the chicken cubes to the bag and toss to coat. You can marinate in the refrigerator for a few hours or use immediately.

- Preheat the oven to 425°F. Place the vegetables on a rimmed baking sheet. Pour the remaining marinade over the vegetables and toss to coat.

- Dump the marinated chicken on the baking sheet, spread evenly, and bake until the chicken is no longer pink and the vegetables are cooked, about 25 minutes.

Makes about 6 servings.

Per serving: 289 calories, 5 g fat, 15 g carbohydrates, 3 g fiber, 42 g protein

---

Quickie Chili

1 lb. 95% lean ground beef
1 onion, chopped
1 medium summer squash, chopped
1 clove garlic, minced,
1 tsp. ground cumin
3½ cups vegetable stock

1 can (15 oz.) black beans, rinsed and drained.
½ cup scallions, thinly sliced

- Cook the ground beef in a large saucepan over medium-high heat, breaking it up with a wooden spoon for about 3 minutes.
- Add the onion, squash, garlic, and cumin and cook for 8 minutes, stirring occasionally.
- When the onion is softened, add the vegetable stock and beans. Stir to combine and bring to a boil.
- Reduce the heat to low, cover, and simmer for 15 minutes, stirring occasionally. Top with sliced scallions and serve.

Makes 4 servings.

Per serving: 323 calories, 8 g fat, 28 g carbohydrates, 11 g fiber, 35 g protein

---

Turkey Meat Loaf

1 small onion, peeled and quartered
½ red bell pepper, stemmed and quartered
1 small carrot, peeled and roughly chopped
2 cloves garlic, peeled
1½ lb. ground turkey
½ cup breadcrumbs
¼ cup low-sodium chicken stock
1 egg, beaten
1 Tbsp. Worcestershire sauce
1 Tbsp. low-sodium soy sauce
½ tsp. dried thyme
½ tsp. salt
½ tsp. black pepper

For the glaze:

½ cup organic ketchup
2 Tbsp. brown sugar
2 Tbsp. low-sodium soy sauce
2 Tbsp. apple cider vinegar

- Preheat the oven to 325°F.
- Combine the onion, bell pepper, carrot, and garlic in a food processor and pulse until finely minced.
- Combine the vegetables with the turkey, breadcrumbs, stock, egg, Worcestershire sauce, soy sauce, thyme, salt, and black pepper in a large mixing bowl. Gently mix until all of the ingredients are evenly distributed.
- Dump the meat loaf mixture into a 13" × 9" baking dish and use your hands to form a loaf roughly 9" long and 6" wide. Mix the glaze ingredients together and spread over the meat loaf. Bake for 1 hour, until the glaze has turned a deep shade of red and an instant-read thermometer inserted into the center of the loaf registers 160°F.

Makes 6 servings

Per serving (with glaze): 243 calories, 9 g fat, 16 g carbohydrates, 1 g fiber, 24 g protein

---

Pan-Seared Salmon with Basil

4 wild-caught salmon fillets, ¼ pound each
½ tsp. sea salt
¼ tsp. fresh ground black pepper
1 medium onion, chopped
2 cloves garlic, minced
3 cups grape tomatoes, halved
2 Tbsp. fresh basil, chopped
1 cup dry whole-wheat couscous

- Coat a nonstick skillet with cooking spray and heat over medium-high heat. Sprinkle ¼ tsp. of the sea salt and a pinch of the pepper over the salmon fillets.
- Add the fillets to the skillet and cook, turning once, until the fish is browned and flakes with a fork, about 10 minutes. Transfer to a plate.
- Add the onion, garlic, and tomatoes to the skillet. Cook, stirring occasionally, until softened, about 5 minutes. Remove from heat.
- Stir in the basil with the remaining salt and pepper.

- Cook the couscous according to the package directions. Top the couscous with the salmon and the vegetables.

Makes 4 servings.

Per serving: 350 calories, 13 g fat, 30 g carbohydrates, 5 g fiber, 28 g protein

---

Vegan Red Lentil Soup

3 Tbsp. extra-virgin coconut oil
1 large yellow onion, chopped
4 cloves garlic, minced
4 fingers of fresh turmeric root, peeled and finely chopped
2 large carrots, peeled and diced
1 Tbsp. ground cumin
2 tsp. garam masala
1 tsp. kosher salt
½ tsp. freshly ground black pepper
½ tsp. chili powder
1 small can tomato paste
1 32-oz. carton reduced sodium chicken broth
2 cups water
1½ cups red lentils, picked over
1 8-oz. package of fresh baby spinach
Zest and juice of 1 lemon

- Heat the coconut oil over medium high heat in a Dutch oven.
- Add the chopped onion, garlic, turmeric root, and carrots. Sauté until softened but not browned.
- Add the cumin, garam masala, salt, pepper, chili powder, and tomato paste. Stir together to work the tomato paste into the other ingredients and sauté for 2 more minutes.
- Add the broth, water, and red lentils and simmer for approximately 45 minutes or until the lentils are tender.
- Five minutes before serving, stir in the spinach and the zest and juice of the lemon. Adjust seasoning with salt and pepper if necessary.

Makes 6 servings

Per serving: 328 calories, 8 g fat, 47 g carbs, 19 g fiber, 19 g protein

South of the Border Stir Fry

2 Tbsp. extra-virgin olive oil, divided
16 oz. turkey breast, cut into bite-size pieces
1 cup onion, chopped
3 cloves garlic, minced
1 can (7 oz.) chopped green chilies, drained
1 orange or yellow bell pepper, chopped
1 jalapeño pepper, seeded and chopped
½ cup tomato sauce
1 tsp. chili powder
1 Tbsp. fresh cilantro, chopped
½ cup brown rice

- Heat 1 tablespoon of olive oil in a large nonstick skillet. Add the turkey and sauté until cooked, about 8 minutes.
- Remove the turkey from the pan to a plate. Add the remaining tablespoon of olive oil to the pan and mix in the onion, garlic, chilies, bell pepper, jalapeño, tomato sauce, and chili powder. Cook over medium heat, stirring, for 6 minutes or until the onions are soft.
- Add the turkey back to the pan and top with the cilantro. Simmer for 3 minutes. Serve over ½ cup brown rice.

Makes 4 servings.
Per serving: 335 calories, 16 g fat, 18 g carbohydrates, 4 g fiber, 30 g protein

Portobello Turkey Burger and Bruschetta with Strawberry Pecan Salad

8 oz. ground turkey
½ tsp. garlic powder
¼ tsp. kosher salt
¼ tsp. black pepper
4 large portobello mushroom caps (stems removed)
2 Tbsp. balsamic vinegar
1 Tbsp. red onion, chopped
2 basil leaves, thinly sliced

2 plum tomatoes, chopped
1 oz. mozzarella, sliced

- In a bowl, mix the turkey, garlic powder, salt, and pepper. Form the seasoned turkey into burger patties.
- Lightly oil a grill or grill pan and heat to medium-high heat.
- Cook the burgers and the mushroom caps, about 4 minutes per side, until the burger is cooked and the portobellos are tender.
- To make the bruschetta, mix together the vinegar, onion, basil, and tomato. Add salt and pepper to taste.
- Place each burger on a mushroom cap, top with a mozzarella slice and bruschetta mixture, and use the remaining mushrooms as "bun" tops.

Makes 2 servings.

Per serving: 260 calories, 12 g fat, 13 g carbohydrates, 3 g fiber, 30 g protein

---

Strawberry Pecan Salad

2 Tbsp. balsamic vinegar
1 tsp. raw honey
¼ cup olive oil
Salt to taste
3 cups baby spinach
1 cup strawberries, sliced
¼ cup pecan halves

- Mix the balsamic vinegar and honey together in a bowl.
- Whisk in the olive oil; add salt if desired.
- Divide the spinach onto four plates. Top with the strawberries and pecans. Drizzle the balsamic vinaigrette on top.

Makes 4 servings.

Per serving: 176 calories, 16 g fat, 9 g carbohydrates, 3 g fiber, 2 g protein

Beef Stew

¼ cup all-purpose flour
1 tsp. salt
½ tsp. freshly ground black pepper
1½ pounds lean stewing beef cut into 1½-in. cubes
2 Tbsp. vegetable oil
2 onions, chopped
3 cloves garlic, minced
1 tsp. dried marjoram
1 tsp. dried thyme
1 bay leaf
1 cup red wine
3 Tbsp. tomato paste
3 cups reduced-sodium beef broth
5 large carrots
2 stalks celery
5 potatoes (about 1½ pounds)
12 ounces fresh green beans
⅓ cup chopped fresh parsley

- Combine the flour, salt, pepper, and beef in a large zip-top plastic bag and shake to coat. Transfer the beef to a plate and save the leftover flour mixture.
- In a Dutch oven, heat 1 tablespoon of vegetable oil over medium heat. Add the beef in batches, adding more oil as needed during cooking until the meat is browned all around. Transfer each batch to a plate when finished.
- Reduce the head to medium-low. Add the onions, garlic, marjoram, thyme, bay leaf, and the rest of the of the flour mixture to the pan. Cook, stirring often, until the onions are soft, about 4 minutes. Add the red wine and tomato paste to the pan and stir with a wooden spoon.
- Put the beef back into the pan along with the broth. Bring to a boil, stirring often, until slightly thickened. Reduce the heat to medium low, cover and simmer for an hour, stirring occasionally.
- Cut the carrots and celery into 1½-inch pieces. Peel and quarter the

potatoes. After the stew has cooked for an hour, add the vegetables to the Dutch oven. Cover and simmer for 30 minutes.

- Trim the ends of the beans and cut them in half. Add the beans to the pan and stir. Cover and simmer for 30 more minutes. Remove the bay leaf and add the parsley. Season with salt and pepper to taste.

Makes 6 servings.

Per serving: 362 calories, 12 g fat, 35 g carbohydrate, 5 g fiber, 27 g protein

---

Pesto Chicken Sandwich

4 whole-wheat tortillas (6" diameter)
¼ cup jarred pesto sauce
½ pound sliced cooked chicken breast, warmed
¼ tsp. salt
¼ tsp. ground black pepper
2 jarred roasted red bell peppers (2 oz.), drained and halved
4 thin slices (4 oz.) mozzarella cheese
4 romaine lettuce leaves

- Preheat the oven to 350°F. Arrange the tortillas on a baking sheet.
- Spread the pesto evenly over each.
- Arrange the chicken slices in a row down the center of each tortilla and sprinkle with the salt and black pepper.
- Top with the roasted peppers and mozzarella.
- Bake just until heated through and the cheese melts.
- Top with the lettuce, roll into a cylinder, and serve.

Makes 4 servings.

Per serving: 328 calories, 16 g fat, 23 g carbohydrates, 3 g fiber, 29 g protein

CHAPTER

10

70 More Delicious Smoothie Recipes

Breakfast Smoothies

Place contents in blender and blend until smooth unless otherwise indicated.

Black and Blue Breakfast

1 cup low-fat milk
1 frozen banana
½ cup frozen blackberries and blueberries
¼ cup old-fashioned oats
1 Tbsp. no-added-sugar peanut butter

Makes 1 serving.

The Belly Filler

½ zucchini, peeled and chopped
¼ cup cooked rolled oats
1 Tbsp. flaxseeds
2 Tbsp. walnut pieces
½ cup unsweetened almond milk
1 scoop plant-based plain protein powder
Water to blend

Makes 1 serving.

Peanut Brittle

1 Tbsp. chunky peanut butter
2 scoops vanilla plant-based protein powder
1 Tbsp. instant sugar-free butterscotch pudding mix
¾ cup fat-free milk
6 ice cubes

Makes 1 serving.

Strawberries and Quinoa

2 cups strawberries, fresh or frozen
1 cup vanilla Greek yogurt
½ cup quinoa, cooked and cooled
2 Tbsp. local honey
1 medium banana
1 Tbsp. chia seeds
1 Tbsp. wheat germ
1½ cups vanilla almond milk

Makes 2 servings.

Peanut Butter Cup

1 cup low-fat vanilla Greek yogurt
½ cup almond milk
½ cup mini semi-sweet chocolate chips
3 Tbsp. Jif Peanut Powder
½ banana
4 graham crackers, crushed
½ cup ice

Makes 2 servings.

Oat Berry

½ cup old-fashioned rolled oats
1 cup 2% milk (more as needed)
½ cup frozen blackberries
2 Tbsp. local honey
¼ cup plain Greek yogurt
2 Tbsp. whey protein powder
¼ cup ice

Makes 2 servings.

Walnut Brownie

1 cup unsweetened chocolate almond milk
1 frozen banana
1 Tbsp. almond butter
2 dates
1 Tbsp. unsweetened cocoa powder
4 ice cubes
1 Tbsp. walnut pieces for garnish

Makes 1 serving.

Creamsicle #1

1 navel orange, peeled, quartered
¼ cup plain Greek yogurt
1 Tbsp. unflavored whey protein powder
2 Tbsp. frozen orange juice concentrate
¼ tsp. vanilla extract
4 ice cubes

Makes 1 serving.

A Berry Cherry Breakfast

1 cup frozen raspberries
¾ cup chilled unsweetened rice milk
¼ cup frozen pitted unsweetened cherries
1½ Tbsp. honey
2 tsp. finely grated fresh ginger
1 tsp. ground flaxseed
2 tsp. fresh lemon juice

Makes 2 servings.

Raspberry Cheesecake

1 cup Greek vanilla yogurt
1 cup frozen raspberries
½ cut vanilla almond milk
1 frozen banana
2 oz. cream cheese

Makes 2 servings.

Green Smoothies

Great for your afternoon smoothie snack.

Sweet Baby Kale

2 handfuls of baby kale
1 cucumber
1 cup cold water
1 cup frozen strawberries
4 dried figs
1 Tbsp. chia seeds

Makes 1 serving.

Vegan Special

3 cups frozen kale leaves
1 rib celery
1 avocado, chopped
¼ cup Italian parsley
½ cup frozen blueberries
1 cup coconut milk

Makes 2 servings.

Strawberry Olive Oil Smoothie

1 cup frozen strawberries
½ cucumber, peeled
1 tsp. vanilla extract
1 Tbsp. extra-virgin olive oil

Makes 1 serving.

Citrus Ginger Spinach

½ cup frozen mango chunks
1 handful baby spinach
¼ cup Greek yogurt
3 Tbsp. orange juice
1 Tbsp. lemon juice
1 1-in. piece of ginger, peeled
½ avocado
¼ cup water

Makes 1 serving.

Green Hornet

¼ cup water
½ cup spinach
2 stalks celery, chopped
½ banana
½ lemon
½ pear
¼ tsp. cayenne pepper

Makes 1 serving.

Romaine Holiday

1 cup romaine lettuce, chopped
½ cup spinach
½ red delicious apple with peel, seeded, and quartered
½ cup unsweetened almond milk
1 scoop plain whey protein powder
1 Tbsp. chia seeds
Water to blend (optional)

Makes 1 serving.

Celery and Kiwi

1 rib celery, chopped
2 large kiwifruits, peeled and chopped
1 cup chopped kale
½ cup fresh orange juice
½ cup cilantro
2 ice cubes

Makes 1 serving.

Green Tangerine Detox

1¼ cups chopped kale leaves, tough ribs removed
2 medium ribs celery, chopped
¼ cup chopped flat-leaf parsley
¼ cup chopped fresh mint
1 cup fresh-squeezed tangerine juice
1¼ cups frozen cubed mango

Makes 2 servings.

Green Grass

½ frozen banana
½ pear
¼ avocado
½ cup baby spinach, loosely packed
½ cup no-sugar-added apple juice
¼ cup water
1 scoop plain plant-based protein powder
Water to blend

Makes 1 serving.

Kale and Hearty

1 cup kale, tightly packed
Handful of cilantro
½ pear
½ avocado
½ cucumber
Juice of ½ lemon
½ -in. ginger, peeled
½ cup coconut water
1 scoop plant-based protein powder
Water to blend

Makes 1 serving.

The Gazpacho You Eat with a Straw

Handful kale leaves, stems removed
1 rib celery, chopped
2 Tbsp. lime juice
½ cup plain Greek yogurt
¼ tsp. ground cumin
1 cup diced tomatoes
1 small English cucumber, chopped
Hot sauce to taste
¼ cup water
½ cup ice

Makes 2 servings.

Strawberry Beet

1 cup frozen strawberries, chopped
1 frozen banana
½ cup coconut water
1 medium beet, scrubbed, ends trimmed, roughly chopped
1 Tbsp. coconut oil

Makes 1 serving.

Smoothie Bowls

Acai Almond Smoothie Bowl

3½ oz. frozen acai pulp
½ large frozen banana
1 scoop vegan protein powder
¼ cup unsweetened almond milk
½ cup frozen mixed tropical fruit or berries

Toppings:

2 Tbsp. almond butter
1 Tbsp. granola
2 Tbsp. fresh berries
2 Tbsp. coconut flakes

Makes 2 servings.

Apple Sunflower Bowl

½ cup skim milk
6 oz. vanilla Greek yogurt
1 tsp. apple pie spice
1 apple, peeled and chopped
2 Tbsp. cashew butter
5 ice cubes

Toppings:

⅓ cup sunflower seeds
½ graham cracker, crumbled (optional)

Makes 2 servings.

Choc Bowl o' Nuts

½ frozen banana
1 fresh banana
1 cup plain Greek yogurt
1 Tbsp. peanut butter
1 Tbsp. almond butter
1 Tbsp. cacao powder

Toppings:

Strawberries
Cacao nibs
Chia seeds
Pomegranate seeds
Semisweet chocolate chips
Sliced almonds

Makes 2 servings.

Blood Sugar Stabilizing Smoothies

The Diabetes 'Beeter'

Beets are nutrient dense and contain a substance called betaine that's particularly effective at turning off the genes responsible for insulin resistance and belly fat storage.

1 medium beet, cooked
1 tsp. coconut oil
1 Tbsp. almond butter
½ cup unsweetened almond milk
1 scoop plant-based plain protein powder

Makes 1 serving.

Fiber Power

1 medium frozen banana
½ cup peaches, fresh or frozen
1 Tbsp. liquid coconut oil
8 oz. orange juice
1 tsp. psyllium husk fiber powder
1 scoop unsweetened whey protein
2 ice cubes

Makes 1 serving.

Avocado Oil, Spinach, and Yogurt

2 Tbsp. avocado oil
½ cup plain Greek yogurt
1 medium banana
10 oz. cold water
2 cups baby spinach, loosely packed

Makes 2 servings.

Spice Root Smoothie

½ cup fresh pineapple, cut into chunks
½ frozen banana
1 Tbsp. turmeric
1 cup unsweetened almond milk
1 scoop plant-based plain protein powder

Makes 1 serving.

The Green Banana

1 ripe banana
½ cup green tea
½ cup milk
1 Tbsp. peanut butter or almond butter
1 Tbsp. local honey
1 cup ice

Creamsicle #2

4 Clementines, peeled
½ frozen banana
½ cup almond milk
5 ice cubes
Dash kosher salt
¼ tsp. vanilla extract
1 tsp. local honey
¼ tsp. ground turmeric

Makes 2 servings.

You'll Love Olive It

1 Tbsp. extra virgin olive oil
1½ frozen ripe bananas, chopped
½ cup frozen blueberries
1 handful of spinach
1½ cups coconut milk
1 Tbsp. almond butter
1 Tbsp. flaxseeds
1 Tbsp. cacao powder

Makes 1 serving.

Immune-Boosting Smoothies

Hawaii 5-Oh!

2 cups seedless watermelon chunks
1 cup mango, cut into chunks
½ frozen banana
1 ice cube
2 tsp. local honey
1 tsp. fresh lime juice
½ tsp. freshly grated ginger

- Puree the watermelon and pour into a glass. Put aside. Blend the rest of the ingredients, pour into glasses and top with pureed watermelon.

Makes 2 servings.

Bloody Martha

1 small tomato, diced
¼ cup cucumber
2 squeezes lemon juice
1 sprig parsley
1 pinch of cilantro
1 scoop plant-based plain protein powder
Hot sauce to taste

Makes 1 serving.

Ginger Kiwi

2 kiwifruits, peeled
1 pear, chopped
1 small zucchini, chopped
1 ½-in. piece ginger
3 Tbsp. cashews

Makes 1 serving.

Green Tea, Blueberry, and Banana

½ cup brewed green tea
2 tsp. local honey
1½ cups frozen blueberries
½ banana
½ cup vanilla soy milk

Makes 1 serving.

Honey Mango

¼ cup mango cubes
¼ cup mashed ripe avocado
½ cup mango juice
¼ cup fat-free vanilla yogurt
1 scoop vanilla-flavored whey protein powder
1 Tbsp. freshly squeezed lime juice
1 tsp. Manuka honey or local raw honey
6 ice cubes
Slice of mango to garnish
Water to blend

Makes 1 serving.

Citrus and Soy

1 cup soy milk
6 oz. lemon-flavored yogurt
1 medium orange, peeled and sectioned
Handful of ice cubes
1 Tbsp. flaxseed oil

- Blend all ingredients except the flaxseed oil. Put into a glass and then mix in the oil.

Makes 1 serving.

Very Berry

1 cup frozen mixed berries
½ cup low-fat plain yogurt
½ cup orange juice
1 Tbsp. shredded coconut to top

Makes 2 servings.

Pomegranate Grape

2 handfuls baby kale
½ cup seedless red grapes
½ cup pomegranate juice
½ cup frozen blueberries
1 frozen banana
½ cup sliced strawberries

Makes 1 serving.

Bahama Daiquiri

½ cup 1% milk
2 Tbsp. plain Greek yogurt
¼ cup frozen orange juice concentrate
½ frozen banana
¼ cup sliced strawberries
½ cup mango, cubed
1 Tbsp. vanilla whey protein powder
3 ice cubes

Makes 2 servings.

Strawberry Kiwi

½ cup cold apple cider
½ ripe banana, sliced
½ kiwifruit, sliced
2 frozen strawberries
2 tsp. chia seeds
1½ tsp. honey

Makes 1 serving.

Dessert Smoothies

Sweeter smoothies for occasional desserts and snacks.

Berries and Papaya

¾ cup frozen strawberries
¾ cup frozen papaya
½ cup 2% milk
½ cup green tea
1 Tbsp. fresh mint

Makes 1 serving.

Grilled Peaches 'n' Cream

Grilling caramelizes the peach flesh, adding a sweet complexity to this creamy smoothie.

1 Tbsp. coconut oil
1 Tbsp. honey
4 peaches, pitted and halved
1 cup vanilla bean frozen yogurt
¼ cup unsweetened almond milk

- While heating a grill, whisk the coconut oil and honey together. Place the peach halves on a plate and brush each peach, front and back, with the coconut oil–honey marinade.
- Grill the peaches flesh side down for 3 minutes or until the fruit caramelizes. Flip and grill the other side for 2 minutes.
- After the peaches cool, add them to a blender with the rest of the ingredients and blend until smooth.

Makes 2 servings.

Key Lime Pie

½ cup fat-free cottage cheese
1 scoop vanilla whey protein powder
1 Tbsp. lime juice
1 Tbsp. local honey
Handful of baby spinach
½ tsp. xanthan gum
5 ice cubes
Water to thin if too thick

Topping:

½ graham cracker, crumbled

Makes 1 serving.

Tastes Like Ice Cream

1 medium frozen banana
¼ cup Greek Yogurt
1 Tbsp. almond butter
½ cup blackberries

- Puree the frozen banana in a blender. In a medium bowl, mix together the Greek yogurt and the almond butter. In a dessert bowl, spoon in alternating layers of the banana puree and then the yogurt-almond butter mixture. Top with blackberries.

Makes 1 serving.

Halloween Frappe

½ frozen banana
⅓ cup pumpkin puree
¼ tsp. pumpkin spice
1 tsp. flaxseeds
1 cup unsweetened almond milk
1 scoop plant-based plain protein powder

Makes 1 serving.

The Girl Scout

¾ cup nonfat Greek yogurt
¼ cup fresh mint, tightly packed
1 cup almond milk
¼ cup dark chocolate chips
1 large handful baby spinach
1 tablespoon maple syrup
6 ice cubes

Makes 2 servings.

Carrot Cake Shake

1 carrot, finely chopped
1 cup almond milk
1 frozen banana
1 Tbsp. local honey
½ Tbsp. ground flaxseed
1 tsp. ground cinnamon
1 tsp. pure vanilla extract
¼ tsp. ground nutmeg
¼ tsp. ground ginger
½ cup ice cubes
Coconut flakes, to garnish
Chopped pecans, toasted to garnish

Makes 2 servings.

Welcome Sunshine

1 cup frozen mixed berries
1 frozen banana
1 orange, peeled and segmented
6 oz. vanilla Greek yogurt

Makes 1 serving.

Chocolaty Smoothie

Chocolate Pudding for Dessert

1½ cups cold nonfat milk
½ package Jell-O instant sugar-free chocolate pudding mix
¾ cups vanilla ice cream
1 scoop plant-based chocolate-flavored protein powder

Makes 2 servings.

Peppermint Pattie

1 large frozen banana
1 cup cashew milk
2-3 large ice cubes
1 scoop chocolate whey protein powder
2 Tbsp. cocoa powder
1 Tbsp. dark chocolate nibs
Pinch sea salt
¼ tsp. peppermint extract

Makes 1 serving.

Choco-Cherry Blizzard

1 cup unsweetened almond milk
½ cup plain Greek yogurt
1 cup frozen cherries
1 Tbsp. chocolate whey protein powder
1 Tbsp. dark cocoa nibs
2 ice cubes

Makes 1 serving.

Chocolate Raspberry

½ cup chocolate-flavored almond milk
6 oz. vanilla Greek yogurt
¼ cup dark chocolate chips
1 cup frozen raspberries or 1 cup fresh raspberries and 4 ice cubes

Makes 1 serving.

Chocolate Chunks

1 banana
3 Tbsp. chunky peanut butter
3 Tbsp. cocoa powder
½ cup of almond milk
Whipped cream for topping

Makes 1 serving.

Dates and Chocolate

1 medium frozen banana
1 cup chopped strawberries
½ medium avocado
4 pitted Medjool dates
1 cup almond milk
1 Tbsp. local honey
2 Tbsp. raw cocoa powder

Makes 1 serving.

Fat-Burning Smoothies

Apples 'n' Cinnamon Spice

½ Honey Crisp apple, chopped
1 Tbsp. apple cider vinegar
½ tsp. cinnamon
¼ cup coconut water
½ cup plain Greek yogurt
1 tsp. vanilla extract
4 ice cubes

Makes 2 servings.

Anti-Inflammation Elixir

2 carrots, chopped
½ frozen banana
½ Tbsp fresh ginger
¼ tsp. turmeric
1 Tbsp. lemon juice
1 cup water
½ cup unsweetened almond milk
1 scoop plant-based plain protein powder
¼ tsp. cayenne pepper (optional)

Makes 2 servings.

The Happy Pineapple

1 cup frozen pineapple
½ cup Greek yogurt, plain
½ cup 2% milk
½ cup green tea

Makes 2 servings.

Tropical Spice

1 avocado
2 Tbsp. lemon juice
½ cup coconut water
1 scoop whey protein powder
¼ tsp. cayenne
1 2-in. piece of fresh ginger
1 cup frozen mango

Makes 2 servings.

A Matcha Made in Heaven

1 cup light coconut milk
1 cup pineapple juice
1 frozen banana
1 tsp. matcha green tea powder
4 ice cubes

Makes 2 servings.

All Red Already

¼ red bell pepper
½ cooked beet
½ tomato
1 celery stick
1 dash cayenne pepper
½ cup unsweetened almond milk
1 scoop plain plant-based protein powder

Makes 1 serving.

Tirami-Smooth

¾ cup part-skim ricotta cheese
2 Tbsp. low-fat plain yogurt
1 Tbsp. slivered almonds
1 scoop chocolate whey protein powder
2 tsp. ground flaxseed
2 tsp. finely ground instant coffee
6 ice cubes

Makes 2 servings.

Chai and Mighty

¼ cup unsweetened almond milk
¼ cup chai tea, brewed from a teabag and chilled
½ scoop plant-based vanilla protein powder
½ frozen banana
½ tsp. ground cinnamon
½ Tbsp. unsalted natural almond butter
Water to blend (optional)

Makes 1 serving.

Harvest Moon

½ cooked sweet potato, cooled, peeled
½ tsp. nutmeg
1 tsp. cinnamon
1 tsp. thyme
1 tsp. basil
½ cup Earl Grey tea, brewed and cooled
1 scoop plain whey protein powder

Makes 1 serving.

Apple Flax

¼ frozen banana
½ large apple with peel, quartered and seeded
½ cup unsweetened almond milk
1 tsp. flaxseed oil
A few dashes of ground cinnamon
1 scoop vanilla plant-based protein powder
Water to blend (optional)

Makes 1 serving.

Coco-Nana Almond Smoothie

1 frozen banana
½ cup plain Greek yogurt
3 Tbsp. almond butter
½ cup coconut water
1 scoop whey protein powder
1 Tbsp. hulled hemp seeds
1 cup ice

Makes 2 servings.

Mr. Nibs

2 bananas, frozen
½ cup almond butter
½ cup light coconut milk
½ cup almond milk
2 Tbsp. heavy cream
½ tsp. ground cinnamon

Makes 2 servings.

Peaches 'n' Cream Oatmeal

½ cup whole milk
½ cup plain Greek yogurt
½ cup rolled oats
1 cup frozen peaches
½ frozen banana
½ cup ice

Makes 2 servings.

The Bee's Knees

1 cup almond milk
1 cup frozen blueberries
1 Tbsp. bee pollen
1 Tbsp. coconut oil
1 tsp. local honey
½ banana

Makes 1 serving.

CHAPTER

11

Frequently Asked Questions

Why is the diet only seven days long?

WHEN IT COMES to starting to establish healthier eating and exercising habits, seven days is ideal: A week is not too long, not too short. We've found that most people can commit to almost anything challenging for a week. These seven days will teach you to become more aware of your hunger and satisfy it with proteins and high-volume, low-calorie whole foods. You won't feel as if you are sacrificing anything. You won't suffer headaches or feel fatigued. And you won't get bored. You will lose weight quickly, which will motivate you to continue on the path of healthy eating and regular exercise.

What do I do after the seven days are finished?

Continue to use smoothies as satisfying low-calorie meal replacements and snacks to keep your cravings at bay and your blood sugar stable. Substitute a high-protein breakfast of eggs, Canadian bacon, and whole-wheat toast for your morning smoothie when you have the time to cook. Your dinners should be similar to those you prepared during the 7-Day Smoothie Diet: high in lean protein, filling, low-calorie vegetables, and a small amount of whole grains. Try our selection of lunch and dinner recipes in Chapter 9. Enjoy berries and whipped cream for dessert, a simple piece of whole fruit, or a dessert smoothie. Go out for dinner occasionally. Just make a habit of choosing wisely and bringing half of your meal home for tomorrow's lunch. Remember that restaurants serve huge portions. Also, continue to eliminate all beverages with added sugars from your diet. You don't need anything but water, flavored waters, unsweetened tea and coffee—and smoothies. And if you find that you've experienced a string of days when your foods were, let's say, less than mindfully chosen, plug in your blender and let nutritious smoothies guide you back on track.

Is the 7-Day Smoothie Diet safe for everyone?

It is important to talk with your physician before starting any diet or fitness program that significantly changes your normal routine. On the 7-Day Smoothie Diet plan, you'll be eating mostly smoothies, plants, and lean proteins, which are all nutritious and healthful, so it's unlikely that you will experience any problems. But check with your doctor nonetheless. Exercise is another story, especially if you have been sedentary. While the "Get Moving!" suggestions in this book are beginner-level, some are rigorous. We always recommend seeing your doctor for a checkup before starting any new fitness regimen.

Should I weigh myself every day?

Try it. If it helps to motivate you, keep it up. Several recent studies have shown that the practice can be effective. In one two-year study of 162 overweight and obese people, those who weighed themselves daily and charted their results dropped significantly more pounds (and kept them off) compared to those who didn't track their weight. But if adding that daily task to your to-do list drives you crazy, don't bother. Hopping on the scale once a week should be enough to give you a sense of how you are managing your weight loss. But do it at the same time during the day in the same state of undress to get the most useful and accurate information. Better yet, stay off the scale and instead pay attention to the fit of your clothing.

I've been doing walking workouts with friends for several years, and I'm not losing more weight. What can I do to burn more calories?

Here are two suggestions:

Keep a three-day food log to get an accurate picture of what and how much you are eating. Exercise can make you hungry. Often, people will underestimate the number of calories they are consuming in a day and overestimate how intense their workouts are.

Mix up your workouts. Our muscles can get accustomed to the same exercise routine over time. By trying some new activities, you can "shock" your muscles into burning more calories. Try strength training, biking, or swimming for a change. Or increase the intensity of your walking. Walk fast for as long as you can and then slow down. Do a walk-run workout. Halfway through your workout, stop and do 10 jumping jacks, 10 jump squats, and 10 push-ups to increase the intensity of your workout.

Can I have sugar and non-dairy creamer in my coffee?

Acquiring a taste for unsweetened coffee and tea is pretty easy; you can accomplish that in about seven days. So please do without the sweet stuff, and that goes for artificial sweeteners, too. It's worth the effort, because it will help you become far less reliant on sweeteners (natural or added) in other foods as well. Without any fiber in coffee or tea, drinking them sweetened is like swallowing a teaspoon (or two) of sugar granules. It goes right into your bloodstream. A little non-dairy creamer is fine if you are lactose intolerant.

What are the best seeds to use in smoothies?

Chia seeds, hemp seeds, ground sunflower seeds, and flaxseed are all great sources of good fats and fiber. We like ground flaxseed because it's easier to absorb. You can buy a one-pound bag for only about five dollars.

Some of my friends have cut back on eating fruit because they say it's too high in sugar. Why are you using fruit in the smoothie recipes?

It's true that there's sugar (fructose) in fruit, as much as 20 grams of it. But there's a difference between strawberries and strawberry ice cream. "It's key to look at added sugars differently than sugar in fruit, because in fruit we're getting so much more nutrition [compared to refined sugar]," says Isabel Smith, RD, a nutritionist in New York City. Fresh, whole fruit delivers antioxidants, minerals, cancer-fighting phytochemicals, water, and fiber.

If I feel hungry before lunch even though I had my breakfast smoothie, can I have a small snack?

First try to distract yourself using one of the Cravings Crusher techniques in Chapter 6. We think you'll find that will help. Also try sipping a cup of herbal tea or a tall glass of ice water with lemon to quell the hunger pangs. After this brief seven-day program, you can add in a midmorning snack. For example, a small organic apple with a spread of almond butter provides fiber, fat, protein, and natural sugar to fill your tummy and provide a burst of energy to carry you through to lunch.

At the end of the 7-Day Smoothie Diet, is it okay to have sugar-free desserts?

There's no benefit to eating foods made with artificial sweeteners, only a downside. Because these sweeteners are so sweet, your brain thinks your body is getting a big dose of sugar. It responds by releasing insulin, which triggers fat storage, just as it would if you had eaten a big bowl of natural ice cream.

My friends use supergreens and superfruits powders in their smoothies. But I found them to be very expensive at health food stores. Are they worth the price?

Fresh spinach, beet greens, parsley, kale, or Swiss chard and fruits like kiwi and papaya will provide all the antioxidant vitamins you need without the unpronounceable fillers that you find in some of those powders. You pay for the convenience of the powders.

Can I make my smoothie the night before?

Sure. When busy, make a batch of smoothies and pour them in wide-mouthed plastic water bottles or glass containers with good lids and store them in the refrigerator. They keep for up to two days, which is very convenient. But there's nothing like a freshly blended smoothie, so try to minimize refrigeration time.

Is "raw" sugar any better for you than white sugar?

Nope. That tawny sugar that comes in those little brown packets is the same as the white stuff: 4 grams of carbohydrate and 16 calories per teaspoon. The only difference is the color. Further processing would turn it white.

I know that most sports drinks are high in sugars and calories. What can I drink after a workout that's not water? I need some flavor!

Try watermelon juice. This flavorful, low-sugar juice is a great natural workout recovery drink, rich in antioxidants and an amino acid that may reduce muscle soreness. Here's how to make it: Cut up 2 cups of seedless watermelon and place it in a covered bowl in the refrigerator to chill for an hour or two. Then put the watermelon chunks into a blender, add a squeeze of lime juice from a quarter of a lime, and puree. If you don't like the pulp, strain the mixture through a fine sieve.

Why are natural sugars better than added sugars? Isn't all sugar, sugar?

You're right. All sugars, whether they come from the bowl on the table, an apple, or a chocolate chip cookie, break down similarly in your body. All sugars impact your blood sugar levels. But when you consume those natural sugars found in fruits and vegetables, you also get a lot of good stuff that you don't get from added sugars. Like what? Like vitamins and minerals, and fiber.

Can I eat power bars for snacks on this plan?

Most energy bars are full of, well, energy, meaning they are high in calories and often loaded with sugars. So we don't recommend them. During the 7-Day Smoothie Diet, smoothies will be your breakfast meal and your afternoon snack of choice. After the week is up, you can substitute in a low-carbohydrate, high-protein bar as a snack as long as you check the nutrition label. You'll want to keep your total grams of added sugars for the day under 25 grams, so be aware of how many grams you are consuming. We think you'd be better off focusing on eating clean as much as possible and filling up on lean proteins and high-fiber, high-water-content vegetables

Call me crazy, but I love to have instant oatmeal for lunch. It's so convenient when I don't have time to go out or order in at work. How can I make it more nutritious?

You're crazy! And really smart! Oatmeal is quick, high in filling fiber, and can be accompanied with so many things that boost the nutritional value—and flavor. If you haven't tried this yet, add in nuts, chia seeds, flaxseed, pumpkin seeds, and sunflower seeds. Mix in fresh blueberries, strawberries, kiwi, peaches, or banana. Boost the level of satisfying protein by mixing in some chocolate-flavored plant-based protein powder.

CHAPTER

12

33 Best Weight-Loss Secrets

WHEN YOU TRAVEL, you probably do some research before you head to the airport or get behind the wheel of your car. If you're going someplace you haven't been before, you probably ask friends who've been to your destination for the inside scoop on the off-the-beaten path sites to see, the best cafes, the hidden-gem restaurants where the locals go, the coolest shops. Hints and tips like these make your visit easier, less intimidating, more efficient, less expensive, and more enjoyable. Armed with that knowledge, you feel better prepared and more enthused for the adventure.

Starting a weight-loss program can be a little like taking a trip to a foreign place, too. Naturally, there are unknowns and the small anxieties they trigger. That's where tips and hints from someone who has been there can help.

Here are some that will help you navigate the 7-Day Smoothie Diet. These are nuggets of advice, tricks, tips, and suggestions that we've found helpful when using smoothies to lose or maintain weight and establish a healthier pattern of eating.

1. Take baby steps. Remember what we said in the beginning of the book about climbing a mountain: You need good hiking boots and stronger legs. You don't climb a mountain without preparation. The 7-Day Smoothie Diet has a built-in warm-up plan of mini goals that take you to the top.

Step one is gathering supplies for making your weight-loss smoothies. You'll need a blender. Use what you have at home. Don't go out and buy one. Eventually, you may want to invest in a high-speed blender like a Vitamix, Smeg, Breville, or KitchenAid. Step two is shopping for protein powder, fruits, vegetables, and yogurt. You can't make smoothies without the goods. Review Chapter 4 for the best ingredients.

2. Have a plan. Choosing which smoothie recipes you'll use for the 7-Day Smoothie Diet before you go shopping will ensure that you have every ingredient you need and help you avoid waste.

3. Drink more water and tea. Drinking smoothies as meal replacements doesn't cover your daily liquid requirements. We'd like to see you consume about 64 ounces of water each day. Remember, some of that water can come from foods, especially vegetables and fruits. Tea and coffee contribute, but beware of the calorie hit you can take if you add lumps of sugar or teaspoons of creamer. Brewed green, white, or black teas are packed with compounds called catechins, belly-fat crusaders that blast belly fat by revving the metabolism, increasing the release of fat from fat cells, and speeding up the liver's fat-burning capacity. In a recent study, participants who combined a daily habit of four to five cups of green tea with 25 minutes of exercise (or 180 minutes a week), lost two more pounds than the non–tea-drinking exercisers. Even tea without sweating offers weight loss benefits by boosting the body's ability to metabolize fat. A study in the *Chinese Journal of Integrative Medicine* found that participants who regularly sipped oolong tea lost a pound a week, without doing anything else to change their diet or exercise habits.

4. Practice living by the 80/20 rule. Eating healthy most of the time and allowing indulgences every once in a while, known as the 80/20 rule, is a lifestyle you can maintain forever. This means that 80 percent of the time, you eat lots of fresh fruits and veggies, whole grains, lean protein, and healthy fats, and that you cut down on the sugar, processed foods, and alcohol. Then, 20 percent of the time, you get the green light to enjoy some chocolate, a glass of wine, or some French fries. Knowing you can indulge a little satisfies cravings so you never feel deprived.

5. Clean your kitchen. Even before you stock up on smoothie ingredients, give your kitchen a clean sweep. In other words, get rid of calorie-dense, high-sugar processed foods. If they are lying around on the counter or in a cabinet that's easily accessed, you will be tempted to eat them, especially when you are bored. Don't create additional temptation for yourself. Bag the snacks.

6. Don't starve yourself. Skipping meals tends to backfire on you. You become so hungry that you lose all willpower and consume the closest, most calorie-dense food you can find, eat too fast, and overeat. Instead, be mindful of your hunger. Satisfy it with a smoothie or high-fiber snack like cut-up vegetables or a high-protein snack like a hard-boiled egg, cheese stick, or a handful of nuts and seeds.

7. Sprinkle on some vinegar. Adding a few tablespoons of vinegar on a sandwich or salad can slow the body's absorption of carbohydrates and reduce feelings of hunger so you eat less. Studies have shown that vinegar taken with a carb-heavy meal can reduce blood sugar spikes by a quarter or more.

8. Eat more fiber. If you hate counting calories and despise eliminating dessert, try this no-brainer weight-loss trick: Simply eat at least 30 grams of fiber daily. University of Massachusetts Medical School researchers found that this technique fuels weight loss and improves health even more effectively than some more complicated diet approaches did. Researchers say that focusing on eating more of a certain nutrient is often easier than eliminating a food for some people. See chapter 13 for some of the best high-fiber foods. Gain a bonus benefit. By eating more fiber, you'll have more regular bowel movements, a sign of good health.

9. Walk, don't sit. While your eating habits have a greater influence on weight gain or loss than exercise will, don't forget the powerful benefits of moving more every day. When you are physically active, your body metabolizes food more efficiently, you build muscle, you sleep better, and you feel happier. All of these can affect your weight loss. So be sure to get at least 30 minutes of physical activity a day. Start by taking the stairs instead of the elevator. According to a University of New Mexico Health Sciences Center study, a person who weighs 150 pounds could lose about six pounds per year just by climbing up two flights of stairs daily.

10. Add oats to ground turkey. Oats are not just a breakfast staple. Gain the heart-healthy, diabetes-busting benefits by making turkey-and-oat meatballs. Add ¾ cup of quick-cooking oats to 1½ pounds of ground lean turkey. Include ½ cup chopped onion, 1 egg, and ½ cup tomato sauce. Roll into meatballs and bake in a pan at 400°F. for 20 minutes. Serve with tomato sauce.

11. Brown bag it. Pack your lunch to take to work every day and you will avoid the temptation of calorie-dense fast-food restaurant options. A study in the journal *Obesity* analyzed the receipts of nearly 8,000 people from 11 different fast-food chains and found that the average restaurant lunch topped 820 calories, and 34 percent of meals purchased had more than 1,000 calories in them. Brining a healthy lunch to work could save you thousands of calories per week.

12. Wrap it right. Instead of using a carb-heavy ten-inch wrap for your next homemade sandwich, go green with a crisp Bibb lettuce leaf. By putting your chicken or tuna salad or hummus in a lettuce leaf instead of a wrap or bread, you'll save at least 150 calories and more than 30 grams of carbohydrates.

13. Go topless. Here's an easy way to instantly cut 70 to 120 calories out of your diet without even noticing: Take the top off your sandwich. Making your sandwich open-face style, with just one slice of whole-grain bread, keeps calories off your plate and allows you to pile on the nutritious toppings.

14. Add chia seeds to your smoothie. We're a big fans of chia seeds because they plump up in liquid, which means they fill you up without loading you down with calories. Plus, they're full of heart-healthy omega-3s, fiber, protein, and calcium. Use them in smoothies or mix them into cottage cheese or yogurt with a handful of blueberries.

15. Make your own hummus. Many commercial hummus tubs are jam-packed with waist-widening additives. To avoid the unnecessary ingredients, whip up your own hummus at home and use it as a dip for crunchy veggies such as carrots and celery. The spread's main ingredient—chickpeas—contains satiating fiber and protein to keep hunger pangs at bay.

16. Use smaller bowls and plates. If you poured your favorite breakfast cereal into a large bowl and a small bowl, we can almost guarantee that you'll put more in the larger bowl. Why? Because a larger bowl makes the food look smaller. You mistakenly think you aren't getting enough, so you keep on pouring. Similarly, the smaller plate or bowl makes your food look much larger, tricking you into taking a smaller portion. In one study, campers who were given larger bowls served themselves and consumed 16 percent more cereal than those given smaller bowls. Swapping dinner plates for salad plates will help you eat more reasonable portions, which can help reduce calorie consumption.

17. Woof it. Get a dog and hoof it. Studies suggest that people who own dogs are healthier and fitter than those who don't, because walking a dog is good forced daily exercise. You'll burn 61 calories in just 15 minutes of walking a dog, according to the American College of Sports Medicine.

18. Have a Happy Meal. If you must have a cheeseburger and fries, indulge, but order the kids' size meal. The smaller portion will satisfy your cravings without undoing the progress you've made on the 7-Day Smoothie Diet.

19. Make Sunday prep day. Prepping healthy, homemade meals can help you avoid hitting up the drive-thru or reaching for convenient processed foods that will cause you to pack on the pounds. Cooking more at home will save you money as well as calories. While cooking dinner on Sunday afternoon, whip up another meal or two to freeze for later in the week. Sure, it takes more time, but it will save you more time when the busy work week starts.

20. Eat mindfully. What's that? Well, let's look at the flip side: The opposite of eating mindfully is eating without thinking. It's consuming whatever is handy or delicious-looking without paying attention to content or portion control. Think of mindlessly chomping through a bag of chips while watching television or rhythmically dipping your hand into a bowl of yogurt-covered peanuts while chatting with a friend at the kitchen table. When you eat mindfully, you pay attention. You pause before you munch. You evaluate your hunger cues and make a smart plan for satisfying them. You make a better choice by selecting a food that's good for you and will satisfy your hunger and your taste buds without triggering blood sugar spikes. Studies in the *American Journal of Clinical Nutrition* found that paying attention while eating helps people lose weight. Distracted eating, by contrast, can lead to overeating by hundreds of calories.

21. Become a label reader. One of the best ways to practice mindful eating is to become a student of the nutrition facts panel on packaged foods. By regularly perusing the nutrition label (and don't forget the ingredients list!), you'll be more likely to make smarter food choices. You'll be amazed at how often you will put a product back on the supermarket shelf after reading unpronounceable things on the ingredients list.

22. Make a guiltless snack. Toss chickpeas with olive oil, spices, and a sprinkle of sea salt. Spread on a sheet pan and bake for 30 minutes at 400°F.

23. Quit the shame game. In her book *The Naughty Diet,* our friend Melissa Miln interviewed thousands of women about body shaming, and they all said the same thing: "They were sick and tired of feeling bad while trying to be good," she writes. "And here's the secret of all secrets: You don't feel bad about yourself when you get fat. You get fat when you feel bad about yourself." This could be because chronic stress raises levels of the stress hormone cortisol in the body, which can trigger belly fat storage. Try being kinder to yourself, which will reduce stress and help melt the pounds away effortlessly.

24. Buy a fruit bowl. Fill it with fruits and fresh vegetables. You're more likely to grab fruits and veggies over less healthy options if they're ready to eat and in plain sight. Katie Cavuto, MS, RD, the dietitian for the Philadelphia Phillies and Flyers, suggests keeping washed and prepared veggies like cucumbers, peppers, sugar snap peas, and carrots in the front of the fridge so they aren't overlooked. Bananas, apples, pears, and oranges should be kept on the counter where everyone can see them.

25. Get comfortable with being boring. Many dieticians and weight-loss coaches advise their clients to limit themselves to just a couple of go-to breakfasts or snacks. Why? Repetition builds rhythm. You don't have to ask yourself, "Hmm, what shall I have?" If you know of a few things that you love that are also low in calories and high in nutrients, why keep searching? Switch things up every couple of weeks, but keep variety to a minimum.

26. Use the half-plate rule. This is another no-brainer way to make weight-loss easy: Fill at least half of your lunch and dinner plate with vegetables. Vegetables will fill you up and keep you satisfied longer than starches, like rice, will because they are high in satiating fiber and water.

27. Suck on a mint. Want to keep from spooning yourself seconds of that casserole or taking an extra chocolate chip cookie? Pop an Altoid in your mouth. We often yearn for more of what we just ate because the taste of the food still lingers in our mouth. So cleanse your palate with a mint or a breath strip and you'll reduce the urge to keep noshing.

28. Send the basket back. We're talking about the bread basket they bring to the table before you order or the tortilla chips and salsa they serve in a Mexican restaurant.

Both are carb-heavy calorie bombs. Ask your server to take them away, and you'll immediately improve the nutritional profile of your restaurant meal.

29. An easier way to catch fish. You'll end up eating more fish with brain-healthy omega-3 fats if you keep your pantry stocked with canned tuna and salmon. Choose light tuna, which contains fewer calories and less sodium. The best canned fish is salmon because it contains fewer toxins like mercury and more of the omega-3s DHA and EPA than other canned fish.

30. Swap in some 'shrooms. If you substituted low-energy-density foods like mushrooms for high-energy-density foods such as hamburger just once a week, you'd save more than 20,000 calories and roughly 1,500 grams of fat over the course of a year without changing anything else about your diet, according to researchers at Johns Hopkins Weight Management Center.

31. Go to sleep earlier to wake up earlier. According to researchers, late sleepers—defined as those who wake up around 10:45 a.m.—consume 248 more calories during the day, as well as half as many fruits and vegetables and twice the amount fast food as those who set their alarm earlier. If these findings sound troubling to you night owls, try setting your alarm clock 15 minutes earlier each day until you're getting out of bed at a more reasonable hour. This may take a week or so but it really works.

32. Push breakfast back. Instead of gobbling down breakfast at home, eat at your desk a few hours later than you typically do. Pushing back your first meal of the day naturally reduces your "eating window"—the number of hours you spend each day grazing. Why is that beneficial? Sticking to a smaller eating window may help you lose weight, even if you eat more food throughout the day, a study published in the journal *Cell Metabolism* found. To come to this finding, researchers put groups of mice on a high-fat, high-calorie diet for 100 days. Half of them were allowed to nibble throughout the night and day on a healthy, controlled diet while the others only had access to food for eight hours, but could eat whatever they wanted. Oddly enough, the fasting mice stayed lean while the mice who noshed around the clock became obese—even though both groups consumed the same number of calories.

33. Make a list. Think writing a grocery list before heading to the store is a waste of time? As it turns out, it may be the key to finally losing weight. A *Journal of Nutrition Education and Behavior* study of more than 1,300 people discovered that shoppers who regularly wrote grocery lists also purchased healthier foods and had lower body mass indexes than those who didn't put pen to paper before heading to the store. Researchers hypothesize that shopping lists keep us organized, which in turn helps us fend off diet-derailing impulse buys (hello, candy aisle). Before heading to the supermarket to stock up, spend a few minutes taking inventory of your kitchen, and then write a list. Be sure to organize it by category to prevent zigzagging all over the place; that ups the odds you'll walk by—and purchase—tempting treats that could derail your weight loss success.

CHAPTER

13

50 Foods That Heal

SOME TIME AROUND 431 B.C., perhaps while he was eating a fig or a few grapes, the Greek physician Hippocrates famously wrote, "Let food be thy medicine and medicine be thy food." It has taken the rest of us a while to recognize that wisdom. But we're starting to come around. Scientific research in recent years has identified important chemicals, primarily in plants, with powerful healing properties.

"We have evidence that we could eliminate 80 percent of chronic disease by eating the right foods," says David Katz, MD, founder of the True Health Initiative and director of Yale University's Prevention Research Center.

That means you can be your own best health care provider even without having gone to med school. So grab a grocery cart and start hunting and gathering your way to a better body. Fill your plate with these superfoods and cure your health problems deliciously.

Foods That Fight Inflammation

If you eat a lot of fried foods, refined flours and sugars, hormone- and antibiotic-laden animal products, synthetic sweeteners, and artificial food additives, your body will begin to transition into a state of chronic inflammation. This inflammatory, high-energy diet builds belly fat, reduces levels of gut-healthy probiotics, induces weight gain, causes joint pain, bloating, and fatigue, and has been connected with a host of diseases, from diabetes and obesity to heart disease and cancer. These foods fight the flames.

Blueberries

A study in the *Journal of Nutrition* showed that eating berries daily could significantly reduce inflammation. Another study in the same journal found that fruit-based drinks could neutralize the inflammatory effects of high-fat, high-

BEST INFECTION FIGHTER: MUSHROOMS

They are a rich source of selenium, which boosts white blood cell production, improving the body's ability to fight infection.

carb meals. Why is this exactly? Well, berries contain a class of antioxidants called flavonoids, but it's the anthocyanins, specifically, that contribute their anti-inflammatory effects by effectively turning off inflammatory and immune genes. And when it comes to anthocyanins, blueberries are king. On top of that, blueberries are rich in vitamin C and another polyphenol, resveratrol, which have both been found to promote anti-inflammatory responses through decreasing inflammatory free radicals.

Tart Cherries

Tart cherries and their juice are high in anti-inflammatory antioxidants. In one study, women who drank tart cherry juice twice a day for three weeks had significantly fewer inflammation markers than women who drank a sugary fruit-flavored drink.

Green Tea

Green tea's inflammation-dousing benefits stem from catechins, the group of antioxidants concentrated in the leaves of tea plants. The most powerful of all catechins, a compound called epigallocatechin gallate, or EGCG, is found almost exclusively in green tea. Scientific studies, like one in the *Journal of Advanced Pharmaceutical Technology & Research*, suggest that the high EGCG and polyphenol content in green tea make it a stronger anti-inflammatory elixir than other teas like black tea. These anti-inflammatory properties have also been credited with preventing the development and growth of skin tumors.

Red Peppers

Peppers are an anti-inflammatory superfood—but go red

to reap the most benefits. Out of the three colors of bell pepper, red peppers have the highest amount of inflammatory-biomarker-reducing vitamin C along with the bioflavonoids beta-carotene, quercetin, and luteolin, according to research in the *Journal of Food Science*. Luteolin has been found to neutralize free radicals and reduce inflammation. Beta-carotene is a carotenoid, a fat-soluble compound associated with a reduction in a wide range of cancers, as well as reduced risk and severity of inflammatory conditions such as asthma and rheumatoid arthritis.

Turmeric

You can thank curcumin for turmeric's beautifully bright, yellowy-orange color—but that's not all it's good for. This active compound has been found to contain potent anti-inflammatory and antioxidant properties. Studies have shown curcumin directly inhibits the activation of inflammatory pathways by shutting off production of two pro-inflammatory enzymes, COX-2 and 5-LOX. For this

BEST CANCER FIGHTER:
BROCCOLI

If cancer is a giant, complex circuit board, broccoli is like the big red OFF switch. The average American eats more than four pounds of the vegetable a year, according to the National Agricultural Statistics Service. And that's a good thing, because there's significant evidence of the value of cruciferous vegetables like broccoli in cancer prevention. In fact, clinical trials show eating steamed broccoli just a few times a week can lower rates of prostate, breast, lung, and skin cancers. Researchers attribute the anti-cancer properties primarily to sulforaphane, a compound that works on a genetic level to effectively "switch off" cancer genes, leading to the targeted death of cancer cells and slowing of disease progression.

HEALING SMOOTHIE

The Flame Cooler (for inflammation)

Studies suggest that tart cherries (not maraschinos!) may be the anti-inflammatory medication of the fruit world. Consider this research in the *Journal of International Society of Sports Nutrition*, which followed 54 healthy runners as they prepared for long-distance runs: Runners who were given tart cherry juice to drink while training reported less pain and soreness than runners who were given a placebo cherry drink.

¾ cup tart cherry juice
1 cup frozen pineapple
½ cup baby spinach
½ cup nonfat Greek yogurt
Water to blend (optional)

Makes 1 serving.

Per serving: 263 calories, 1 g fat, 53 g carbohydrates, 3 g fiber, 15 g protein

BEST TUMMY TAMER:
GINGER

One of the most surefire ways to soothe an upset tummy is with ginger—a remedy that's been used since ancient times. "Its properties naturally relax the intestinal walls," says Dr. Susan Albers, a clinical psychologist at the Cleveland Clinic. "Try a cleansing light broth with ginger and shredded chicken or carrots, or sip a homemade ginger tea."

reason, curcumin has contributed to a range of beneficial health effects: preventing cognitive decline, liver damage, and heart disease, easing joint inflammation and pain associated with arthritis.

Nuts

Although not as strong as the animal-based omega-3s, DHA and EPA, nuts (particularly walnuts) are a great source of a plant-based anti-inflammatory omega-3 known as ALA. Almonds are one of the best sources of antioxidant vitamin E, which helps protect cells from oxidative damage (a byproduct of inflammation), and hazelnuts contain the highest amount of immunoprotective oleic acid.

Canned Light White Tuna

According to a 2016 study published in the *American Journal of Clinical Nutrition*, the most effective omega-3 when it comes to reducing specific markers of inflammation is DHA over EPA. So how do you get more of the powerful fat into your diet? It's easy (and cheap)—just grab a can of light skipjack tuna, which is one of the best sources of the bioactive fatty acid.

BEST VISION PRESERVER:

COOKED KALE OR SPINACH

The National Institutes of Health found that people who consume the most lutein—an antioxidant pigment found most potently in leafy greens like spinach and kale—are 43 percent less likely to develop macular degeneration. The lutein becomes more easily absorbed if you cook the greens beforehand.

Foods That Boost Brainpower

According to the Alzheimer's Association, Alzheimer's disease—a neurodegenerative disorder that is the most common type of dementia—disproportionately affects women more than men, and is currently the fifth leading cause of death in females. In fact, almost two-thirds of Americans with Alzheimer's are women, but many experts attribute the disparity to the fact that women often live longer than men, and old age is the greatest risk factor for Alzheimer's. Experts suspect other risk factors to be related to the decrease in consumption of antioxidant-rich foods, which typically scavenge cell-damaging free radicals, which may lead to cognitive decline.

Shrimp

Shrimp are the most potent source of an essential and hard-to-get nutrient called choline. This neurotransmitter building block is necessary for the structure and function of all cells, and a deficiency in this compound has been linked to neurological disorders and decreased cognitive function.

BEST BLOAT BLOCKER:

YOGURT

One and a half cups of live culture yogurt (with healthy gut bacteria) encourages good digestion and pushes food through the digestive system. The beneficial bugs also help reduce gas and bloating that can occur from eating beans and dairy products.

Not only does it act as brain food, but it can also help lower your risk of breast cancer.

Cinnamon

There's a genetic basis to Alzheimer's, and if the disease runs in your family, it's especially important to make changes to your lifestyle to minimize your risk. One of those changes is adding cinnamon to your diet. The same constituents of cinnamon that moderate spikes in blood sugar levels—proanthocyanidins and cinnamaldehyde—exhibit other properties that can inhibit the formation of protein aggregates that cause Alzeheimer's, according to a study in the *Journal of Alzheimer's Disease.*

Almond Butter

Swapping peanut butter for almond butter might better your chances of beating age-related memory loss. Almonds contain high concentrations of vitamin E (three times more than peanut butter), which has been shown to help reduce the risk of cognitive impairment. And some studies indicate the nutrient can also slow the decline caused by Alzheimer's disease. For a snack, spread a teaspoon over celery, or mix a spoonful into your morning oatmeal.

HONEY, I SHRANK A1C

Honey has a less dramatic impact on your blood-sugar levels than regular sugar does. Plus, unlike table sugar, it's packed with beneficial compounds.

HEALING SMOOTHIE

The Nutty Professor (for brain health)

Blend up some noggin nourishment by tossing walnuts into your next smoothie. A study in the *Journal of Nutrition, Health and Aging* found that people over 60 years old who consumed about 6 to 7 walnut halves a day performed better on tests of memory, concentration, and the speed of processing information. Walnuts are rich in brain-boosting, mood-lifting omega-3 fatty acids, the plant-based version of famed fish oil.

½ banana
1 tsp. dark chocolate morsels (dairy free)
1 cup unsweetened almond milk
⅛ cup chopped walnuts
6 ice cubes
⅓ cup chocolate plant-based protein powder
Water to blend (optional)

- Add all of the ingredients to the blender in the order listed. Blend on high for at least 2 minutes or until smooth (note: this may take longer if your blender isn't very strong). Scrape down the sides of the blender. Add a few tablespoons of water if it's too thick. Blend again.

Makes 1 serving.
Per serving: 229 calories, 11 g fat, 26 g carbohydrates, 7 g fiber, 28 g protein

Foods That Lower Blood Pressure

Apples

In addition to the 4.5 grams of blood pressure–lowering fiber you'll get from each apple, you'll also enjoy a healthy helping of quercetin, which has been deemed an effective antihypertensive, according to the results of a study conducted at the University Complutense of Madrid's School of Medicine.

Arugula

This peppery-flavored leafy green contains some of the greatest amounts of nitrates of any food. This is key, because nitrates are converted into nitric oxide, an important signaling molecule in the body that acts as a potent vasodilator to relax the arteries, reducing blood pressure and improving circulation. It also keeps the endothelial cells lining the arteries healthy and supple.

Low-Fat Yogurt

A study of more than 2,000 adults revealed that those who consume just 2 percent of their total daily calories from yogurt have a lower incidence of hypertension than those who eat the creamy stuff less often. And some yogurts deliver a nice dose of potassium, a proven blood-pressure reducer.

Dark Chocolate

A little dark chocolate can go a long way when it comes to

HEALING SMOOTHIE

Blueberry-Banana Crème (to lower blood pressure)

Powerful antioxidants called anthocyanins found in blueberries may trigger the production of nitric oxide in the body. Nitric oxide is a key compound that relaxes blood vessels so they widen and improve blood flow, which helps to lower blood pressure. In a study in the *Journal of the Academy of Nutrition and Dietetics*, researchers found that postmenopausal women with high blood pressure who consumed a daily dose of freeze-dried blueberry powder (equivalent to 1 cup of fresh blueberries) for 8 weeks experienced a 5 percent decrease in systolic blood pressure and a 6 percent decrease in diastolic blood pressure. And their NO levels increased 69 percent! Just say, "yes" to this NO-boosting smoothie.

1 cup frozen blueberries
1 ripe banana
1 cup plain nonfat yogurt
1 cup packed baby spinach

Makes 1 serving.

Per serving: 153 calories, 0.5 g fat, 32 g carbohydrates, 4 g fiber, 7 g protein lowering those numbers, thanks to its flavonoid content. Flavonoids, a type of plant-based pigment, have been linked to reduction in blood pressure, thanks to their ability to improve endothelial function, according to researchers at the University of Manitoba. Just make sure you're choosing real dark chocolate for the biggest benefit; foods high in sugar, like most milk chocolate bars, have been linked to an increase in blood pressure by researchers at New Zealand's University of Otago.

GOOD NIGHT, SWEET TART

If you're having trouble falling asleep, count on fruit instead of sheep. Recent research shows that a glass of tart cherry juice twice a day can help some people sleep about ninety minutes longer per night. Researchers say it's due to the natural melatonin in tart cherries.

Sweet Potatoes

Indulge your carb cravings and lower your blood pressure at the same time by whipping up a batch of oven-baked sweet potato fries tonight. Sweet potatoes are a good source of hypertension-fighting resistant starch and vitamin C, as well as being loaded with blood pressure–lowering beta-carotene.

Tomatoes

In addition to boasting plenty of vitamin C and quercetin, tomatoes are a great source of lycopene, which researchers at Ben-Gurion University in Israel have linked to significant reductions in blood pressure.

Foods That Reverse Diabetes

Avocados

Avocados really do live up to their hype. Not only are they creamy, delicious, and versatile, they can help you maintain healthy blood-sugar levels. Avocados contain a significant amount of healthful fats and dietary fiber, which help slow carbohydrate digestion and absorption. Including avocado in meals is a scrumptious way to help prevent spikes in blood sugar.

Oatmeal

"Oats contain a type of fiber called beta-glucan, which seems to have an anti-diabetic effect," explains Jackie Newgent, RDN, CDN, author of *The All-Natural Diabetes Cookbook*. "I advise people with diabetes to steer clear of added sugars by enjoying savory rather than sweet oatmeal."

Lentils

Thanks to its high fiber content, this legume prevents blood sugar spikes by delaying the process of transforming carbo-

BEST ANXIETY SOOTHER:

BANANA

Grab a banana when you feel anxious or stressed out. A medium banana contains about 30 percent of your daily requirement for vitamin B6, which helps your body produce the calming brain chemical serotonin, says Laura Cipullo, RD, a nutritionist and expert in treating eating disorders.

HEALING SMOOTHIE

Mr. Bean (to defeat diabetes)

Beans in a smoothie? Before you gag, realize that the other stuff you dump into the blender—bananas, strawberries, and mint leaves—will mask the flavor and texture of the beans. It's delicious! Now consider how powerful beans and legumes can be in the war against diabetes and you'll understand why we had to find a way to include them in a smoothie. In one study in the journal *Archives of Internal Medicine*, researchers asked 121 adults with type 2 diabetes to eat one cup of beans a day for just three months. When compared with a similar group who ate high-fiber wheat instead of beans, the bean eaters significantly lowered their blood sugar levels. Another study followed 3,000 adults who didn't have type 2 diabetes for more than four years. The participants were asked to replace a half serving of bread, rice, or baked potato with legumes every day. At the end of the trial, researchers found that participants who ate the legumes slashed their risk of developing diabetes significantly compared to people who did not eat beans regularly.

¼ cup kidney beans
½ frozen banana
½ cup frozen strawberries
4 mint leaves
1 cup unsweetened almond milk
¼ scoop plant-based plain protein powder

Makes 1 serving.

Per serving: 340 calories, 4.5 g fat, 53 g carbohydrates, 11 g fiber, 24 g protein hydrates into glucose in the bloodstream. Plus, lentils fill your belly, satisfying your hunger so you don't overeat.

Quinoa

This nutty, trendy whole grain is a good source of fiber and protein, making a smart pick for a diabetes diet, says nutritionist Sarah Koszyk, RDN: "With the fiber and protein combination found in quinoa, you'll feel fuller and have better blood sugar control."

Foods That Lower Cholesterol

Apples

Apple peels are rich in a type of soluble fiber known as pectin—the same fiber added to jams or jellies to thicken them up. Pectin helps your body excrete the bad cholesterol by latching onto it and guides it out of your digestive system.

Oats

Not all carbs will shatter your weight-loss goals. This nutrient-dense, fiber-rich cereal grain is loaded with the cholesterol-lowering soluble fiber beta-glucan. Just 3 grams of beta-glucan has been shown to reduce LDL cholesterol levels from 5 to 10 percent and thus reduce your risk of coronary heart disease. The same fibers that cause your oats to double in size overnight, beta-glucans lower bad choles-

1,000

How many more micronutrients you'll get by eating black raspberries instead of red raspberries.

HEALING SMOOTHIE

PB & Oats (to cut cholesterol)

When you just can't face another bowl of oatmeal in the morning, sow your oats in a blender to get your LDL-cholesterol-lowering fix. Bonus: The fiber in this tasty shake will keep hunger away until lunchtime.

½ cup of oatmeal
2 frozen bananas
1 cup almond milk
½ cup Greek yogurt
⅛ tsp. ground cinnamon
Pinch of nutmeg
Pinch of salt
1 Tbsp. peanut butter
1 tsp. maple syrup

Makes 2 servings.

Per serving: 381 calories, 8 g fat, 65 g carbohydrates, 9 g fiber, 16 g protein

BEST CAVITY STOPPER:
HARD CHEESE

Finish your meals with a hard cheese to ward off cavities. Since it's so chewy, it increases saliva flow, which wards off cavities. Plus, cheese contains calcium and casein, both of which protect against demineralization.

terol by forming a layer in the small intestine that blocks cholesterol from entering your bloodstream, according to a review in the journal *Food & Function.*

Grapefruit

University of Florida researchers found that grapefruit's pectin could lower total cholesterol and drop your ratio of LDL to HDL cholesterol. Consider digging into half a grapefruit before your morning oatmeal or slice a few segments on top of your starter salad.

Flaxseeds and Chia Seeds

One of the hallmarks of a balanced diet is to have a good ratio of omega-3s to omega-6s. A 1:4 ratio is ideal, but the modern American diet is more like 1:20. That leads to inflammation, which can trigger weight gain. One of the easiest ways to upgrade your diet is by sprinkling some ground chia seeds or flaxseed into your overnight oats, on top of baked goods, or mixed into your smoothies. Animal studies suggest a chia-rich diet can lower harmful LDL cholesterol and protect the heart. A recent study in the *Journal of Nutrition* found that when patients who were susceptible to cardiovascular disease ingested just 30 grams (about four tablespoons) of ground flaxseed daily, they could reduce circulating LDL cholesterol levels by 15 percent as quickly as one month.

Foods That Fight Depression

Blue Potatoes

Blue potatoes aren't a common supermarket find, but they're worth looking out for on your next trip to the farmers' market. Blue spuds get their color from anthocyanins, powerful antioxidants that provide neuroprotective benefits like bolstering short-term memory and reducing mood-killing inflammation. Their skins are also loaded with iodine, an essential nutrient that helps regulate your thyroid, staving off exhaustion and depression along the way.

Chamomile Tea

Research shows that chamomile tea not only brings on better sleep but improves your cognitive functioning during the day, too.

Eggs

Eggs are loaded with mood-promoting omega-3 fatty acids, zinc, B vitamins, and iodide, and because they're packed with protein, they'll also keep you full and energized long after you eat them. Need another reason to crack some shells in the morning? A 2008 study in the *International Journal of Obesity* found that people who ate two eggs for breakfast lost significantly more weight than those who chowed down on a bagel.

Halibut

One of the best choices of fish for feeling content and boosting weight loss, a steamed piece of halibut has an impressive amount of protein and affects your serotonin levels.

Milk

Research has shown that people who are low in vitamin D have higher rates of depression and anxiety. It can be difficult to get your vitamin D naturally from sunlight, especially in the winter, which is why you should make an effort to get your fill via fortified foods or a supplement. Many nutritionists suggest working milk fortified with vitamin D into your diet. You can pour it onto your cereal, add it to your smoothies, or use it as a replacement for cream in your cooking.

Mussels

Mussels are loaded with some of the highest naturally-occurring levels of vitamin B12, a vitamin countless adults are missing out on. What's B12's mood-saving trick? It helps insulate your brain cells, keeping your brain sharp as you age. Mussels also contain the trace nutrients zinc, iodine, and selenium, which keep your thyroid—a major mood regulator—on track. Another benefit? Mussels are high in protein and low in fat and calories, making them one of the healthiest, most nutrient-dense seafood options out there.

A PLUM CHOICE

Stone fruits (plums, peaches, and nectarines) may help you avoid metabolic syndrome, a fancy term for the combination of belly fat, high cholesterol, and insulin resistance.

Seaweed

Seaweed is packed with depression-fighting iodine, which isn't always so easy to find in food. Iodine is critical for your thyroid to function properly, which affects your energy, weight, and even your brain function, leaving you feeling blue when you have too little, and a whole lot happier when you're meeting your goals.

Walnuts

You probably already know that nuts are high in heart-healthy unsaturated fats, but when it comes to boosting your mood, you'll want to pay particularly close attention to walnuts. "In addition to healthy fats the magnesium and omega-3 fatty acids found in walnuts have both been shown to positively impact serotonin and dopamine levels (mood hormones)," says Tanya Zuckerbrot, MS, RD, and the founder of the F-Factor Diet. "Balanced levels of serotonin and dopamine may help to prevent clinical depression."

HEALING SMOOTHIE

FLAX TIME (for defeating depression)

Like walnuts, flaxseeds are a top plant source of omega-3 fats, which studies suggest may be helpful in boosting mood and reducing symptoms of depression. Flaxseeds' anti-inflammatory properties also contribute to brain health.

TIP: Grind your flaxseeds before using them in smoothies.

1 Tbsp. ground flaxseed
2 cups fresh baby spinach
1 orange, peeled
1 carrot, peeled
½ banana
½ cup unsweetened Greek yogurt
¼ cup unsweetened almond milk

Makes 1 serving.

Per serving: 326 calories, 4 g fat (0 g saturated), 50 g carbohydrates, 10 g fiber, 27 g protein

Foods That Prevent Cancer

Chickpeas

The main ingredient in hummus can also help you battle cancer. A study published in the journal *Nutrition and Cancer* discovered that chickpeas contain anti-cancer agents called protease inhibitor concentrates.

Cauliflower

When you chop, chew, and digest cauliflower, its glucosinolates break down and form biologically active compounds known as indoles and isothiocyanates. According to the National Cancer Institute, this cancer-preventive duo can deter the development of breast, lung, colon, liver, and stomach cancers.

Citrus Zest

If you love oranges, lemons, and grapefruits, think outside the circle. The rinds of these citrus fruits contain a powerful compound that boosts the body's production of detoxifying enzymes. In fact, consuming zest regularly can help reduce the risk of squamous-cell skin cancer by 30 percent and shrink existing tumors, say University of Arizona researchers. Add citrus zest to salads, vegetable sides, and, of course, smoothies!

DO THE RIPE THING

Which is healthier, red bell peppers or green? Would you believe the red has up to six times as many vitamins and minerals? The reason is that red peppers are left to ripen on the vine, where they absorb all the good stuff from the earth. See red—and go!

HEALING SMOOTHIE

Cauliflower Power (for cancer protection)

Cruciferous vegetables like cauliflower are noted for their anti-cancer qualities. Several studies have linked eating broccoli, cauliflower, cabbage, kale, and other veggies rich in sulfur-containing compounds. to lower risk of cancers of the bladder, breast, stomach, lungs, and colon. Getting your daily dose of cruciferous plants is easy if you use frozen cauliflower "rice," which blends up easily. Try this power shake, which contains other cancer-fighters like vitamins C and K, and folate.

1 cup frozen riced cauliflower
1 cup frozen strawberries
1 frozen banana
¾ cup unsweetened almond milk
1 Tbsp. almond butter
½ avocado
2 tsp. local honey

TIP: Reserve a few strawberry and banana slices for garnish.

Makes 2 servings.

Per serving: 244 calories, 12 g fat, 34 g carbohydrates, 9 g fiber, 5 g protein

Pomegranate

Cracking open a pomegranate is probably one of the best things you can do for your health and flat belly goals. The fiber-rich arils (the edible, bursting seeds in the fruit) can actually help your body inhibit the growth of hormone-dependent breast cancer, a study published in *Cancer Prevention Research* proves. The acid in pomegranates can potentially protect against breast cancer by suppressing estrogen production and preventing the growth of cancer cells. And they're not the only health food staples rich in ellagic acid; raspberries, strawberries, cranberries, walnuts, and pecans are, too.

Milk

A study published in *Cancer Prevention Research* found that vitamin D could reduce breast cancer risk in women by up to 50 percent. And another more recent study associated low levels of vitamin D in the blood with a heightened rate of breast cancer tumor progression.

Spinach

Spinach is a potent source of lutein and zeaxanthin, two carotenoids that have resulted in a 16 percent reduction in the rate of breast cancer if consumed abundantly. This salad green is also rich in DNA-strengthening folate, a B vitamin essential during pregnancy. A study published in the journal *PLoS ONE* linked low levels of folate to an increased breast cancer risk.

Tomatoes

Tomatoes are particularly rich in lycopene, an antioxidant that, unlike most nutrients in fresh produce, increases after cooking and processing. Dozens of studies suggest a relationship between regular intake of lycopene-rich tomatoes and lower risk of prostate, lung, and stomach cancers, skin damage, and cardiovascular disease. Consider splurging on organic. Research suggests organic tomatoes may have higher levels of disease-fighting polyphenols and vitamin C than conventionally grown varieties.

Foods that Prevent Heart Disease

Dark Chocolate

Dozens of studies show that people who consume cocoa—as a hot drink or as dark chocolate—are in much better cardiovascular shape than those who don't. One nine-year study reported in the journal *Circulation Heart Failure* found women who ate one to two servings of high-quality chocolate per week had a 32 percent lower risk of developing heart failure than those who said no to the cocoa. Researchers attribute cocoa's health benefits to its high concentrations of polyphenols and flavanols, anti-inflammatory compounds that help protect the heart. When you're buying it, just make sure to pick up dark chocolate that contains 74 percent or more cocoa solids, as these are the flavanol-rich compounds.

Edamame

The soybean pods are an excellent source of magnesium, folate, and potassium, nutrients that support heart health by lowering blood pressure. Plus, the fiber in edamame protects the heart by boosting the body's ability to produce low-density lipoprotein (LDL) receptors, which act like bouncers, pulling "bad" cholesterol out of the blood. Researchers at the University of Leeds analyzed a number of studies and found that risk of cardiovascular disease was significantly lower for every 7 grams of fiber consumed.

Legumes and Beans

Unlike animal sources of protein, legumes and beans are free of unhealthy fats. That might be the very reason one study found that people who consumed legumes at least four times a week had a 22 percent lower risk of heart disease compared with those who consumed them less than once a week. Equally encouraging results were published in the *Canadian Medical Association Journal.* A scientific review of 26 clinical trials discovered that eating ¾ cup of beans daily could reduce levels of "bad" cholesterol in the blood by 5 percent.

Olive Oil

A study in the *New England Journal of Medicine* found that the Mediterranean diet, which includes healthy fats like olive oil, prevents about 30 percent of heart attacks, strokes, and deaths from heart disease in people at high cardiovascular risk. Olive oil, in particular, is loaded with monounsaturated fats (MUFAs), which lower "bad" LDL cholesterol and raise "good" HDL cholesterol, which helps in lowering your risk of heart disease.

HEALING SMOOTHIE

Turmeric Carrot Blast (for heart health)

Curcumin is the main active ingredient in this orange-yellow spice and it's a powerful antioxidant. In fact, some nutritionists consider it the most effective supplement on the planet. Touted for its medicinal properties for thousands of years, turmeric is particularly important for heart health as an anti-inflammatory that protects blood vessels and arteries from damage. Some studies even suggest that it may be more effective against high cholesterol than traditional statin drugs.

3 carrots
1 orange
½ lemon, juiced
1 tsp. turmeric root powder
1 Tbsp. sunflower seeds
1 cup water
½ cup ice cubes

Makes 2 servings.

Per serving: 100 calories, 3 g fat, 19 g carbohydrates, 5 g fiber, 3 g protein

Salmon

Fatty fish like wild salmon, mackerel, and herring owe their super health-promoting powers to their high omega-3 content. These powerful anti-inflammatory fatty acids can help decrease your odds of dying from heart disease by more than 33 percent, help lower your risk of arthritis, and possibly make your baby smarter.

Sprouted Garlic

"Sprouted" garlic—old garlic bulbs with bright green shoots emerging from the cloves—usually ends up in the garbage. But scientists report that this type of garlic has even more heart-healthy antioxidant activity than the fresh stuff. Aged garlic extract, also known as kyolic garlic or A.G.E. is a popular supplement because it's odorless. A study found that participants who took four pills a day saw a reduction in plaque buildup in the arteries.

Yogurt

The protein- and probiotic-packed base of many smoothies has been found to help control both systolic (the top number) and diastolic (the bottom number) blood pressure thanks to the yogurt's gut-loving bacteria, according to a study published in the *American Journal of Hypertension*. Researchers tested 55,898 female subjects and 18,232 male subjects who suffered from high blood pressure and supplemented their diets with two or more weekly servings of yogurt. At the end of the experiment, findings revealed that the yogurt supplementation decreased the women's cardiovascular disease risk by 17 percent while men's risk was slashed by 21 percent compared to folks who consumed less than one monthly serving of yogurt.